BIG SOBER ENERGY

BEFRIEND YOUR BRAIN. NURTURE YOUR BODY.
EMBRACE YOUR RECOVERY MAGIC.

BIG SOBER ENERGY
BEFRIEND YOUR BRAIN. NURTURE YOUR BODY. EMBRACE YOUR RECOVERY MAGIC.

Author:
Adrienne van der Valk

Title:
Big Sober Energy: Befriend Your Brain. Nurture Your Body. Embrace Your Recovery Magic.

Disclaimer:
The events and conversations in this book have been set down to the best of the author's ability. In some cases, names and details have been changed to protect the privacy of individuals.

Printed:
In the United States of America
First edition January, 2023
ISBN:
9798389171978

Published by Feminist Hotdog Media

www.bigsoberenergy.com

For Evelyn, Thomas, Patrick, and Daniel

BIG SOBER ENERGY
READER BONUSES

This book is for you, and my most sincere wish is that you feel empowered to use it. To make it as simple as possible for you to integrate these energy practices into your life, I've linked helpful resources throughout the book that add scaffolding or offer you the opportunity to deepen your learning.

All resources linked throughout the book are available in one place at **bigsoberenergy.com/reader-bonuses.** Simply enter your email to access the resource landing page. You can bookmark that page and come back to it whenever you need it. (I'll send you the link via email as well.)

This list is a work in progress; I'll keep you updated whenever I improve an existing resource or add something new!

TABLE OF CONTENTS

PART I
THE BEGINNING

CHAPTER 1

"FORMER ALCOHOLIC"

*"Labeling makes the invisible visible, but it's limiting.
Categories are the enemy of connecting. Link, don't rank."*

— GLORIA STEINEM

WHERE TO BEGIN?

The hardest part of telling a story is knowing where to start—especially when you're still living inside the story.

I thought I wanted to begin by telling you about my twisted love affair with alcohol and why and how I eventually quit.

There's no shortage of stories within that story. There was the time I got so drunk at a conference I was presenting at that I had to be half-carried back to my hotel room (thank you, nameless Florida conference-goers) and almost missed my 6:00 am flight home.

Or the time I jumped out of a moving car because I was furious at my boyfriend for reasons I had completely forgotten by the next day.

Or maybe I could tell you about falling down a concrete staircase and the resulting scars that appear like invisible ink blotches on my knees whenever I stay out in the sun too long.

But weaving together scraps of soggy memories doesn't feel like the right place to start. Not because I want to hide my (decades' worth of) messy drinking. Recovery doesn't tidy up the past, and I embrace that. I'll share plenty of anecdotes in the chapters ahead when they're relevant. But messy is not quite the energy I want to bring to the beginning of a book about harnessing and growing your personal power.

The energy I want to bring is *excitement!* It's the beginning of our journey together, and I want to talk about *you*, my new friend!

First of all, I am so excited and grateful that you're here. Even though we don't know each other, you found this book for a reason. I believe we are connected, and I don't take that connection lightly. I will do my best to honor it during our time together.

I'm guessing you're here because you're tired of collecting your own messy drinking stories, and it's time to make a change. Or you've already gotten alcohol out of your life, and you're looking to energize your recovery. Or maybe you were called by something else entirely.

In any case, congratulations! By taking the small action of picking up or downloading this book, you've already shifted the energy in your life toward showing greater care for your body and your spirit.

Showing care for yourself can only benefit you and the people around you!

I'm also assuming that something about the concept of using energy work as a sobriety tool resonates with you. Do you already have a spiritual practice? Or a sense that there's more to this life than meets the eye, and you're ready to start exploring? Whatever your relationship to the concept of energy, there's so much useful information for you in this book.

That's what I can't wait to tell you about—the practices, realizations, and ideas I've learned from various teachers and authors over the years, combined, refined, and adapted for myself and, now, for you. The things that finally allowed me to disembark the Hot Mess Express.

How did I get from jumping out of moving cars to writing a recovery book? We need a place to push off from, and to establish where that is, I want to share a few fork-in-the-road moments that shaped my drinking years, as well as some snapshots of what happened in between.

Together, I hope they'll help you get to know me, how I came to energy work, and how you can save yourself years of trying what *doesn't* work and start incorporating practices that can radically shift your life into recovery gear.

Moment 1: Falling in love.

At age 18, I started binge drinking, and I didn't stop for 24 years. I didn't drink every day, but when I did (which was often), I had no off switch. As they say in AA, one was too many, and a thousand was never enough.

My introduction to alcohol happened in an unremarkable way—Lynchburg lemonades mixed by an older sibling in a friend's basement when her parents were out of town.

It continued in a normal way, too. If college is no longer synonymous with drunkenness (and thank god things seem to be trending in that direction), in the 90s it definitely was. Being plastered multiple days a week was completely acceptable, and in my friend group, it was encouraged. Drinking a lot—and often—was a badge of honor.

It wasn't until I had been out of school for a few years that I began to notice my attachment to drinking, and to my identity as a drinker, was out of the ordinary.

For the people around me, alcohol was like a bonus to whatever we were doing. In my eyes, it was the main attraction. It wasn't uncommon for me to miss plans because I decided to stay holed up in whatever bar we'd chosen to party at before an event or show. I saw absolutely no point in having one glass of anything. Go big or go home was my motto, and I almost never chose home.

I loved alcohol. When I knew I had an opportunity to drink on a given night, I'd think about it all day and feel giddy, like I had a date with a favorite lover. When I met new people, my first curiosity about them was whether or not they drank and how much. When the friends around me slowed their partying and became less available to drink with, I'd simply transition to a new, younger set of friends.

They say people with alcohol use disorder experience arrested development. I sometimes wonder if that's why it was so easy for me to keep my proverbial barstool warm year after year while the cast of characters rotated around me, aging into the party scene, then back out again.

Despite being trapped in the amber of alcohol, I still managed to live a life that seemed functional, even enviable, to people on the outside looking in. I held interesting jobs. I traveled. I earned graduate degrees. I maintained deep and rewarding friendships, even with people I no longer drank with. I played roller derby and became a yoga teacher.

But as I got older, the drinker's badge of honor no longer held the same social shine. My current crew was growing weary of my antics. Missed work days started adding up. Rather than advertising my drinking prowess as I had before, I began avoiding scrutiny, bobbing and weaving like a champion boxer whenever anyone got too close to the truth.

Because I'm a white woman with a middle-class upbringing and a lot of social privileges, I also avoided much of the judgment and many of the consequences that befall people who don't have the same level of privilege, despite my being *truly* shitty in public *many* times.

There are two names often used to describe people like me: "functional alcoholic" and "gray-area drinker." I dislike both these terms because they imply that drinking the way I did is only *marginally* problematic. No hideous rock bottom to report? Cool, nothing to see here.

If you can hold down a job, avoid DUIs, and don't get the shakes every morning, our society basically looks the other way—*even if it is extremely fucking obvious that you have a problem.*

And it's not like our culture is tripping over itself to help or show compassion for the people who *do* lose their jobs and total their cars, particularly if they are poor, Black, or brown. We (the collective we) are very bad at assessing or addressing alcohol use disorder, talking about its many intersecting causes, or even admitting that it influences people in diverse ways that fall along a broad spectrum. We like to put our drinkers into two categories: *okay* and *not okay*.

Passing as okay is hard work, and it got harder as time went on. In my thirties, I became increasingly unpredictable and nasty when I drank. I started having trouble differentiating my dreams from reality. I found evidence on my body of accidents I didn't remember. I lost days to hangovers so brutal I honestly thought I might die. I lost opportunities and the respect of many people I admired.

I existed in this liminal space between "normal" drinker and "obviously an alcoholic, oh my god, why aren't you at an AA meeting right now?" It was lonely and exhausting—and I fought as hard as I possibly could to stay there.

Every once in a while, though, I'd have an experience that was expensive, embarrassing, or dangerous enough that I started sneaking furtive glances at the idea of cutting down or maybe even taking a break.

Moment 2: Admitting I had a problem (kind of).

One day, after waking up to evidence of a particularly ugly and unnecessary fight with my boyfriend, my desperation finally overcame my desire for secrecy. I made an appointment to see a counselor at a treatment center.

Blacking out terrified me. This didn't happen often, but when it did, I *definitely* heard about it the next day. The aggression, the refusal to cooperate when it came time to leave a party or get in a cab, the realization I had called or texted people spewing bullshit, posted embarrassing photos on social media, or—worst of all—*driven*.

I told the counselor all of this. She asked me a few questions and looked at my questionnaire. Then, she told me a long story about her own battle with alcohol and pills before informing me that I needed to check myself into residential treatment.

I stared at her, dumbfounded. Residential? Like for *alcoholics?* No way.

I had a thesis to write, three part-time jobs, and a roller derby team to co-captain. Was I supposed to scrap my whole life because I needed help learning how to control my drinking? *Fuck. That.*

When I told the counselor I was not in a position to seek residential treatment, she said there was nothing else she could do for me. So, I left, tears stinging my eyes. I never sought formal treatment again. I continued to drink for another ten years.

Leaving the treatment center became another major fork-in-the-road moment for me. It bisects my drinking story for two reasons.

One is that—deep down and despite the many passes friends, coworkers, and cops were giving me—I knew the intake counselor was probably right to recommend residential treatment. I was so out of touch with how bad things had gotten that I simply could not hear it. But her certainty freaked me out. It meant I could no longer pretend I didn't have a problem.

The other thing was that it cemented my lack of trust or faith in traditional recovery spaces. It had taken everything in my power to make the appointment with the counselor and to fill out the questionnaire honestly (for the first time ever). Being given one option and one option only backed me into a corner. And, like most animals, being cornered ignited my instinct to *get the fuck out of there.*

I was determined to show the counselor she was wrong, and I did manage to stay sober after that for about three months.

But the thing is:
...if you rely solely on willpower...
...and refuse to tell anyone that you're not drinking...
...or to even acknowledge it's a problem...
...or to do any introspection about why you love alcohol more than yourself...

...or to change anything about your life...
...or where you spend time...
...or who you hang out with...

...it's extremely difficult to stay on the wagon.

You might abstain for a while, but it's a duplicitous, avoidant, white-knuckle-y existence. It's not sustainable. And it's not recovery.

I didn't know any of this at the time. I was too busy hiding the fact that I was trying and failing to quit over and over and *over* with no information and no support. I didn't know about triggers or reward cycles or neural pathways or trauma responses or self-sabotage. The only explanation my broken brain could conjure up was that I was monstrous, flawed, weak, and doomed to drink forever.

Which brings us to another fork-in-the-road moment.

Moment 3: Giving up on giving up.

I had tried and failed so many times to quit drinking. The only evidence my brain could point to was, "Sobriety is impossible for me."

So, I gave up. Instead, I decided to stop obsessing about getting off the alcohol roller coaster altogether and committed to improving my life and my crumbling mental health in other ways. I literally Googled, "How to make your life better," and the self-help universe was happy to answer my call.

The search turned up countless, smiling, mostly white gurus. All had overcome crippling depression, bankruptcy, cancer, or some other life-upending challenge before building mini-empires based on the solutions they had "discovered."

To me, most of their discoveries looked like slightly rearranged versions of the same solutions, but I figured I was in no position to judge. Shoving cynicism aside, I did what they told me. I got up early. I planned my days. I journaled. I said affirmations. I exercised. I made lists of things I was grateful for and visualized my perfect life in vivid detail.

And I continued to drink.

I also started reading like a maniac. My titles of choice were almost exclusively in and adjacent to the genre known as "quit lit."

I read harrowing stories of extreme rock bottoms and research-heavy tomes about the brain science of addiction and inspiring tales of triumph and redemption. (I've included some of my favorites in the resources at the end of this book.)

I learned about what was happening inside my organs (including my brain) every time I drank. (Yikes.)

The stories were rough—and relatable. As I read, it slowly dawned on me that maybe I wasn't a freak or a loser. There were other people like me out there, and they had managed to quit *and chosen to tell other people about it!* This was revolutionary for me.

But I continued to drink.

The other notable thing I did was meditate; specifically, I practiced a form of Buddhist meditation called vipassana or insight meditation. Vipassana invites you to focus on your breath and observe the passing moments exactly as they are without judgment. My sessions only lasted five or ten minutes at first, but I did it every damn day, which is wild because my track record of doing activities that benefited me usually didn't last more than 72 hours. Something changed after my first few morning sessions: the quiet started to feel necessary. I *wanted* to meditate. You might even say I craved it.

I continued to drink, but the experience had shifted.

I started to notice that time slowed down between having an urge to drink and reaching for a bottle. It almost felt as if I were watching myself from across the room. There was a growing disconnect between when a craving hit me and when the earthy tang of red wine hit my tongue. It was as if my rational mind was feeling around for soft spots where it could squeeze in long enough to remind me that alcohol had long ago ceased to be my friend.

Moment 4: October 22, 2018

One night, about three months after I started my self-improvement campaign, I went out to a concert with a friend and obliterated myself on cheap white wine and whatever else we came across that night. (I'll never know because I blacked most of it out.)

The hangover was epic. For three days, I felt like my body had been turned inside out. Waves of anxiety and dread broke over me relentlessly while my heart pounded out of my chest. With every beat, the blood pulsing in my ears felt like it was begging, *"Please stop, please stop..."*

I didn't know it then, but I was in another fork-in-the-road moment. I only knew I had hurt myself—again, badly—and that, for some reason, the not-okay-ness of the experience stuck with me this time. I was disgusted but also sad and worried for myself. I kept reading and meditating.

And, without consciously deciding to, I didn't drink.

After the clouds of pain had cleared and the urge for alcohol crept back in, I found that time had slowed even more. When my vision zeroed in on a wine bottle, the part of my mind I had been feeding with affirmations, data, stories, and uninterrupted silence finally broke through and gently steered me in another direction.

Day after day, and then week after week, I didn't drink.

I had never experienced anything like this before. Previously, my stretches of sobriety were the result of gritted teeth and pure white-knuckle stubbornness, a resource that always petered out in a few days, weeks, or months at the most.

But three months (my longest sober streak to date) came and went. I continued reading and meditating and doing all the things. I even added a new affirmation to my daily collection, one I had never said before because it always felt like a lie: *I do not drink alcohol.*

And I didn't.

I wish I could say that fateful concert was the very last time I drank, but it wasn't. In my first year of sobriety, I had two slips. But unlike previous wagon falls that had left me feeling like a busted-up failure, these incidents revealed that I no longer tolerated the energy alcohol brought into my life.

Rather than feeling familiar in a comforting way, drinking had become a reminder of something I'd let go of and regretted allowing back in— even for a night. The next time booze came calling, the door stayed closed, and it has remained closed ever since.

I'm writing these words almost exactly four years after that last fork in the road. I don't know what the future holds, but for now, I still read and meditate and do all the things.

And I still don't drink.

There's so much more to say—about how I told people, evolved my practices, started feeling feelings I didn't want to feel, found a sober community, and slowly began repairing pieces of my life that had fallen to shreds while I was drinking. But I'll save those stories for the chapters ahead.

---

 *To read a fuller account of my recovery story, visit **bigsoberenergy.com/reader-bonuses**.*

THREE REFLECTIONS

Before we dive in deeper, I want to highlight three reflections that stand out to me from my quitting story. I do my best not to dwell in regret, but these are things I wish I had known, and I want to pass them on in case they can save you even one moment of pain.

1. You don't have to do this alone.

I asked for help exactly once and then struggled for a decade when the conversation didn't turn out the way I wanted. Don't do that. The recovery world can be an odd and sometimes inhospitable place, but it's worth it to persist.

Finding your people in recovery is like landing on a good therapist or finding someone kind and compatible to date. It often doesn't happen on the first try. If I hadn't been so closed off to talking about how drinking was affecting me, I might have checked out a local group, made an inquiry to my insurance company, or reached out to one of the few sober people I knew.

I'm fortunate that I eventually figured things out and found a supportive community. But I believe I could have started my recovery much earlier if I hadn't stubbornly insisted on going it alone. (More about this in Chapter 15.)

2. Not drinking is not recovery.

For me, recovery meant changing the conditions of my life to create space for something other than alcohol.

I don't think it is a coincidence that I finally let go of alcohol *after* I stopped obsessing about it. My time and energy were directed elsewhere, and that place was filled with practices that literally reshaped my brain. The conditions of my life changed because my energy and my mind changed, and alcohol no longer fit me the way it used to.

I still have cravings, but they don't scare me anymore. I understand what they are, why they are happening, and what I can do about them. For me, this understanding has made long-term sobriety much less difficult than I always believed it would be, based on how hard I struggled to stay sober for even a few days at a time. As long as I keep reading and meditating and doing all the things, the chemistry equation in my brain stays relatively balanced, and the conditions remain optimal for sobriety.

This may not be true for everyone, but since so much recovery rhetoric warns us to stay scared of alcohol, to sit in our powerlessness over alcohol, and to avoid being around alcohol—and alcohol, alcohol, *ALCOHOL*—I think it's worth offering a different perspective. What if we didn't put alcohol at the center of our recovery? (More about this in Chapter 4.)

3. *You don't have to label yourself.*

Not knowing how to talk about my drinking kept me from telling other people about my struggle. The only word I knew was *alcoholic*, and I was not willing to go there. In fact, refusing to call myself an alcoholic is what kept me out of AA—that and the fact that I lived in the Deep South and, being more of a witchy type than a Christian, I was pretty sure Jesus would be a barrier between the other group members and me.

Now that I'm open about why I no longer drink and have had opportunities to talk to many other people about their experiences, it's clear to me that I inherited an outdated belief. You do not need to label yourself as an alcoholic to recover.

Many people find comfort in this label and feel strongly that it applies to them. That's great! I am not one of those people, and yet I still needed help. Help should not be held hostage until someone breaks down and calls themselves a word they don't believe they are. There's nothing therapeutic or beneficial about gatekeeping recovery support, in my view. If our goals are the same, why does it matter what we call ourselves?

"Alcoholic" also isn't a very useful term from a medical perspective. Sure, there are diagnostic checklists and tests that measure damage from alcohol use, but they don't offer any real explanation for why someone becomes controlled by their drinking or what kind of treatment will be best for them. Labeling people as alcoholics or addicts doesn't meaningfully distinguish between drinkers who are physically dependent and drinkers who are not. Plus, if you ask multiple doctors what their definition of an alcoholic is, as Catherine Grey did in her wonderful book Sunshine Warm Sober, you will hear multiple and often contradictory answers.

Thankfully, there's a shift happening in some communities toward talking about problem drinking as behavior that falls on a spectrum. I'm hearing more references to *alcohol use disorder* and less black-and-white rhetoric that separates alcoholics from everyone else. But it is a slow shift.

I want to tell you about a recent experience to illustrate why I think *alcoholic* fails as a universally explanatory word.

About a year ago, I signed up for a fancy clinic that offered a "new kind of healthcare" and promised state-of-the-art medical services—the cutting edge of everything.

Before getting sober, going to the doctor was an incredibly stressful experience for me. As I mentioned before, lying on medical intake forms was second nature, but I was always terrified that some test would reveal the truth, that my "2-3 drinks per week" claim was underreported tenfold, and I would be busted.

At my new clinic (which felt like it had been designed by Apple), I was excited to answer the intake questionnaire. I proudly declared zero when the nurse asked about my weekly intake of drinks, explaining that I used to drink a lot but not anymore. She tapped a few letters into her iPad and moved on. That was the extent of the conversation.

It was a little disappointing, to be honest. I was secretly hoping for some validation or at least acknowledgment of this hard thing I had done. But no pat on the back was administered, and there were no follow-up questions.

In fact, I might have thought the nurse overlooked this aspect of the conversation altogether had I not requested my medical records a few months later. As I scanned the health history, my eyes froze on two words that surmised this clinic's only takeaway from my decades-long struggle with drinking: *Former alcoholic.*

Ummm, what?

I had certainly not used the word alcoholic to describe myself. I had not told her how much I drank previously. She had not asked why or how I stopped or what health impacts I had noticed. Labeling me an alcoholic based on the few words spoken in that exchange struck me as downright bizarre.

And *former* alcoholic? Everyone I know who embraces this term is pretty adamant that an alcoholic is an alcoholic for life. Again, I'm not in love with labeling myself as anything for life, but if you're going to use the label, I don't think it works within that worldview to add the word "former" in front of it.

Aside from the weirdness of seeing those words applied to me, I was left feeling pretty unimpressed with my "state-of-the-art" clinic. Sure, it had spaceship examination rooms, but its handling and documentation of that conversation felt like the analysis of someone whose training consisted of watching a few seasons of *Intervention*. *This* is how "cutting-edge" medical professionals talk about addiction?

RECOVERING OUTSIDE THE STATUS QUO

I'm sharing these reflections with you because I want to be clear that recovery work is still a new frontier. We have a long way to go before we understand substance use disorders, how to talk about them, how to treat them, and why some people experience them while others do not.

Yes, there are amazing therapists, practitioners, and treatments out there, but there are also many well-intentioned people who regurgitate outdated and unhelpful ideas. No one knows everything. There's still much ground to be broken.

I don't consider myself in any way a pioneer, but I do represent a voice speaking from outside the status quo of the recovery world.

- I am not a Christian. I was raised Catholic, but for most of my adult life, I was an atheist. Now, my spirituality blends beliefs and practices drawn from animism, Celtic, Buddhist, and Theosophical traditions, and includes relationships with guides, deities, and ancestors.

- I got sober on my own (which, to be clear, I DO NOT recommend).

- I've never attended a 12-step program.

- I believe substance use disorder is a function of a suffering society, not of individual defects or failings.

- And I'm not afraid to speak up when I disagree with how we discuss addiction or treat people who experience it.

What I offer you with this book is my perspective, my stories, and my experience of what worked for me as someone who back-doored my way into recovery. I wrote this book to share my understanding of why sobriety finally arrived and stuck around once I shifted the energetic conditions in my life.

Energy work is how I came to characterize the collection of practices that got me here, and I believe it has a place in the broader conversation about how to treat substance use disorders. I make no promises that what worked for me will work for you, but I believe the practices you'll encounter in this book can help you improve aspects of your life, no matter where you are on your recovery journey.

Every interaction between a book and a reader is a unique alchemical experience. You and I might read the same book and take away completely different messages, creating something entirely different out of the information. I've always thought that was so cool.

Being on the author's side of the experience is exciting but also a little terrifying. Even though I wrote it, *Big Sober Energy* is yours now. No one can predict how you will integrate it or how reading it will impact your life. I have my hopes, of course, but this is an exercise in surrender.

I've kept these trials, triumphs, epiphanies, and ideas inside for years. It's time to let all of that energy out into the world!

By turning the pages of this book, you've already begun engaging in the work—directing your energy toward your intention to learn, grow, and improve your life. I hope you feel a shift beginning to stir. I can't wait to see where it takes you.

CHAPTER 2

HOW TO USE THIS BOOK

"I am always doing that which I cannot do, in order that I may learn how to do it."

— PABLO PICASSO

WHAT IS THIS BOOK?

When I was drinking, I wanted two things.

1. Booze.
2. Someone to tell me how to not want booze anymore.

If you are looking for #2 as well, I wish I could be that someone for you, but you've probably figured out by now that someone doesn't exist.

There are many books and programs out there, some of which promise you "the easy way" to quit drinking. This promise seems reckless to me.

I believe all people can be helped, but no single approach works for all people.

Alcoholics Anonymous is the best-known program for getting sober, offering 12 familiar steps to recovery. The evidence of AA's efficacy is difficult to assess[1], but it's free, people have used it for decades, and many find value in the self-reflection and accountability the steps encourage.

But AA may not be your thing, and you should know there are many other options that offer realistic and evidence-based advice for changing your habits and mindset. These include Smart Recovery, Recovery Dharma, Tempest Sobriety School, The Booze Break Up, The Luckiest Club, Sober Mom Squad, This Naked Mind, Sober Powered, and a growing list of other mentorship and coaching programs (the space I work in).

Most sober people I know—including myself—got and stay sober using a combination of programs, books, groups, spiritual guidance, and medicinal and nutritional support. Discovering the right combination for you takes time and commitment and, unfortunately, cannot be learned from a single book.

Therefore:

> **This is *not* a book about how to get sober.**
>
> **This *is* a book about how to create conditions in your life that will make sobriety easier, more effective, and more enjoyable.**

It's about approaching some of the things you're probably already doing to get (or stay) sober in a new, intentional way.

It's about having a compass to rely on, so you aren't traveling the road of recovery feeling quite so naked.

It's about nurturing instincts for self-preservation that many of us either never developed or neglected until they went dormant.

And, mostly, it's about empowering you to curate a wonderful life that's worth staying sober for.

You are entitled to peace, love, laughter, and joy, even if you fucked up a lot in the past. Intellectually understanding your entitlement is different than believing it or living it emotionally and physically. My hope is that the practices I share will allow you to fully embrace your right to a wonderful life—body, mind, and spirit.

HOW TO GET THE MOST OUT OF THIS BOOK

There's no right or wrong way to read this book, but I want to point out something about the structure. The practices are grouped into three intentionally sequenced sections:

1. navigating yourself

2. navigating other people

3. navigating the world

This sequence is grounded in my belief that establishing trust, boundaries, and compassion for ourselves puts us in a much stronger position to handle (sober—*yikes!*) the challenges inherent in our relationships with other people and the unavoidable realities of the world (warming oceans, pandemics, and all).

Regardless of whether you work through the practices sequentially, I encourage you to try a few from each section. (Chapter 16 offers you guidance about where to start.)

Recovery is a bit like a paint-by-numbers activity. If you *only* work on one part of it, the picture will emerge lopsided or monochromatic. You won't achieve what you set out to achieve. But that doesn't mean you have to follow all the rules. I encourage you to jump around and customize your painting. Color in the eyes first and the face last. Make the sky purple. Your painting doesn't have to look like anyone else's. You do you.

Above all, don't try everything all at once or become paralyzed by all-or-nothing thinking. It would be shocking and, frankly, weird if you adopted every practice in this book. (Full disclosure: *I do not practice everything in this book all the time!*)

Browse, experiment, take what feels useful, push yourself to try what feels needed. Certain practices will resonate at different stages in your recovery journey, so don't be afraid to put this book down and pick it up again periodically. Think of it as a reference, not a checklist.

THE PRACTICES

Most of the practices I've written about include four common elements: intention, meditation, aligned action, and integration.

Four elements may seem like a lot, but over time these will start to become second nature. You won't always have to remember each one individually, and they don't have to take up a lot of time. In fact, once you incorporate these practices into your life, the four elements will cease to feel like individual steps at all. You will find yourself flowing from one to the next, and engaging in them naturally as you move through your day-to-day experiences.

1. Intention

There is no energy mastery without intention.

In Sanskrit, the word for intention is sankalpa, which can also translate to resolution or free will. According to the Eshwar Bhakti collective, in Vedic tradition, a sankalpa is declared "to ourselves and to the God within us" prior to doing spiritual work. It is a tool to "refine the will, and to focus and harmonize the body."

I would like to respectfully make use of this tool in our work together.[2]

We can't get what we want unless we know what that is. For a long time, setting intentions was the hardest part of energy work for me; it felt foreign and somehow selfish to ask myself what I wanted. I was far more inclined to survey what I thought everyone *else* wanted before pursuing any action or outcome.

For people-pleasers, wafflers, and drifters like me, learning to set intentions is the skill that yields the most immediate and radical results because it empowers us to wrangle our scattered energy and drive it toward a destination.

Depending on the context, setting your intention might look like journaling to gain clarity on your desired outcome or exploring subconscious narratives and deciding to replace them. It might also look like a vision, a goal, or a future you want to manifest.

Do yourself a favor and get as specific as possible. What does your intention look like, taste like, and most importantly, feel like? How will you know when you've achieved it?

"Be a good person" is too blurry of a milestone to tangibly pursue.

"Be someone who spends quality time with my nieces and nephews" has a texture (flannel pajamas), a flavor (Sour Patch Kids), a feeling (delighted exhaustion), and usually some very cute photographic evidence.

Your intention is likely to change throughout your recovery. THAT IS A GOOD THING. There's no reason to remain singularly focused on an outcome if it stops making sense or no longer lights up your soul simply because you once thought you wanted it. Consistency can be a gift, but consistency for consistency's sake can hold us back from where we want to go.

2. Meditation

You know from reading my story how I feel about the power of meditation, so I won't belabor that point here. But, I do want to pound the table about two points.

One, regular mindful meditation will magnify the power of any energy work you embark upon. The mental space and self-awareness meditation creates will open both energy channels and new neural pathways that make the previously impossible seem inevitable. It will accelerate your progress and prepare you to conquer any unforeseen potholes (or, more likely, chasms) in the road. It's the missing ingredient that makes *everything* better.

I'm usually the queen of "whatever—you do you!" But when it comes to meditation, I am an unapologetic evangelist. I consider meditation the equivalent of life-saving medication, and I would never, ever, *ever* dream of skipping a dose. I don't care if you make your bed or floss your teeth or work out or compost your vegetable scraps. But for fuck's sake, please do this one thing, OK? I know you don't want to, but do it anyway. Your future self will thank you.

If you're still reading after that diatribe, here's the second point I want to make: Don't let the meditation steps involved in these practices deter you. These should be viewed as mini-meditations, literally a minute or two to center and breathe and prepare yourself.

Meditation in this context is preparation for putting your intention into motion. It's taking a beat to quiet your mind and clear any unhelpful self-talk that might be buzzing in your brain. It does not replace daily meditation, but it extends the benefits of daily meditation by allowing you to connect quickly to yourself by entering a meditative state. Once you do that, you're ready to begin.

3. Aligned Action (and a plug for ritual)

The aligned action step is where the transformation happens. It is the "what" of an energy practice.

There are many different ways of conceptualizing energy and its transformation. The oldest references known to exist come from the Vedic texts upon which Hinduism is based, and many modern references to energy and energy work have Hindu and Buddhist philosophy as their foundations.

Sometimes when I tell people that I use energy work as a tool for recovery, they assume I'm talking about reiki or qigong, both of which focus on healing or moving life force energy within the body. I have found both reiki and qigong beneficial, but I am not an expert in energy healing, nor am I qualified—culturally or academically—to dispense advice about how to engage in these modalities.

So what *do* I mean by aligned action?

The aligned action steps in this book include activities or rituals intended to shift potential—seen and unseen—to meet an outcome or achieve a state of being.

An aligned action may occur within or outside the body, but is not a healing modality in and of itself. As you'll see, many of these steps include physical movement and breathing to deepen and leverage our mind-body connections. Others focus more on mental or practical habit formation. All are focused on harnessing imagination, emotion, and the power of the subconscious mind as a tool of transformation.

Aligned actions do not have to be complicated or time-consuming. You can create one out of anything:

- Placing your hand on your stomach or your heart.
- Connecting to your intuition and allowing it to serve as your guide.
- Asking yourself, "Does this decision move me closer to or further away from the sober life I desire for myself?"
- Washing your hands and envisioning the water cleansing you of anxiety and doubt.

Growing up, I attended a Catholic church every Sunday morning. The smell of incense and the sound of chanting are still deeply embedded in my memories of weekly mass and holy day celebrations. Rituals marked moments of transition and transformation within the service and communicated to everyone seated in those hard-backed wooden pews that what was happening was sacred. Even the act of dressing for church was a form of ritual.

Whether we're aware of them or not, most of us subconsciously engage in daily rituals, from the technique we use to apply makeup to the way we fix our coffee. When we align these acts with our intentions, they become multipliers of our power.

I'm not saying you have to add frankincense and gilded chalices to your daily energy work (unless that's your thing, in which case please be as extra as possible). But if the definition of a ritual is to mark an action as valuable or symbolic of a transformation, then ritualizing our energy work grows both its effectiveness our investment in its meaning.

4. Integration

If you've ever studied yoga with a skilled teacher, you likely spent a few minutes lying quietly on your mat at the end of class. Savasana—or corpse pose—is an opportunity to be still without the expectation that you must do or be or think anything. It is your body and mind's opportunity to simply *be* while passively absorbing the benefits of the work you recently completed. Your heart slows, your skin cools, and your muscles relax. You have permission to observe these sensations without telling yourself a story about what they mean. Savasana is time set aside for you to integrate the experience of an asana (posture) sequence.

Throughout the book, I urge you to build a little savasana-inspired stillness into the conclusion of your recovery practices. Why? Because it is an opportunity to engage in mindfulness on a micro level, to pause and anchor in the feeling of what you've experienced before you rush off to the next thing. To integrate the experience.

Integration isn't only beneficial after a planned practice. It can help you move on from unexpected stressors that might flood your body with adrenaline and cortisol throughout the day.

Say someone screams at you in traffic or your dog gets in a fight or a work call doesn't go the way you thought it would. All three examples may catch you off guard and cause a stress response. Taking a moment at the *conclusion* of such an experience to separate yourself from the stressor and examine how you feel will allow you to reset much more quickly.

Have you ever had a boss who tells you to drop everything and do Task A but then berates you for not completing Task B? This was a weekly occurrence for me earlier in my career (before the word "gaslight" had fully made its way into the lexicon[3]), and the experience would throw me into a tailspin.

I would *obsess* about confronting my boss, pointing out her inconsistencies, listing all the ways I had gone above and beyond to anticipate her needs, only to be chastised for overlooking some detail we'd never discussed. My body remained in a near-constant state of agitation, and I drank excessively every night to try to bring myself back to what felt "normal" to me. Predictably, as soon as I would stop ruminating on one incident, another one would occur.

Fast-forward several years and hundreds of hours of mindfulness training, and my response to being criticized looks very different.

Now, when someone points out a mistake, I listen to comprehend what they are saying, not to immediately defend myself or refute them. I no longer have any investment in being "right" because either a) I did make a mistake and I should own it or b) they are one of those people who find fault in everything, in which case I have little-to-no chance of changing their behavior in that moment.

Next, I feel my feelings, notice *where* I'm feeling them, and take some deep breaths. If I'm rattled, I'll step away and do some stretches, take a walk, or watch a funny video. I separate myself from the experience and remember that I am not my mistake, and this person's anger is about them, not me.

Finally, I reset and move on. If there's meaning to be made from the experience, I give myself time to ponder it. But not everything is a lesson; some things just suck, and we don't have to make them suck more by allowing them to hang around, clouding our consciousness.

Over time, taking this integration step has helped me enormously when responding to stressful experiences or even taking on new challenges. I rarely sweat the small stuff, and I'm much more confident in my capacity to handle the big stuff.

QUICK REFERENCE GUIDES

Now that you have a handle on how the book and the practices are structured, I don't want you to stress about how to keep track of what you learn. Whether you decide to read straight through or skip around, you'll likely want to come back to specific chapters or sections when you need them. To make this easier, I've included some Quick Reference options for you.

Chapter 16 offers you step-by-step instructions for how to make a Getting Started plan based on the shifts you want to make in your recovery. It also offers suggestions for what to do if you experience a slip and feel tempted to hurl your whole body off the wagon (we've all been there!).

Appendix C, Big Sober Energy Resources, lists all the downloadable worksheets and meditations, as well as other resources mentioned throughout the book, so you can find them all in one place.

Appendix D, Chapters at a Glance, is a reference guide to help you quickly access details about the practices you might need without going back through the whole book.

WHY LISTEN TO ME?

Finally, why should you listen to me? I actually suggest that you don't—at least not exclusively.

Yes, I've trained, studied, and coached students in meditation, energy work, and recovery. I'm confident that what I've written is valid, well-researched, and helpful. But my primary suggestion to you—always, about everything—is to *listen to yourself.*

Sure, read what I have to say. Read what other people have to say, too. But don't take any of it as gospel. If you've struggled with substance use disorder, your trust in your judgment is probably diminished. But just because you've got learning to do doesn't mean you are unfit to gauge what feels right in your soul.

Not every piece of recovery or self-help advice is for you (even if the person dispensing the advice assures you it's for *everyone*). Take the practices that resonate with you and leave the rest—for later or for never. You decide.

We hear a lot in recovery circles about needing to suppress our egos because, otherwise, we'll carry on acting like we're invincible and never take responsibility for our dependency or our actions.

But, in my experience, primarily working with people raised as women, egos aren't the problem; it's usually the opposite. Many of us have absorbed messages that we're flawed or weak our entire lives. Alcohol offers a way to feel brave and whole for a few hours. It's an absolute champion at that. But, in sobriety, we must learn to be our own champions, and that means believing that we can be more than OK—we can be *great!*—without alcohol. Suppressing our egos is a barrier to that important project.

Learning to trust and believe yourself again is its own form of energy work. That's why the very first practice I write and teach about is noticing how you feel without immediately rushing to change it. Your feelings are there for a reason. Befriending them—even the icky ones—will serve you well.

But before you attempt any of these practices, ask yourself this question: Do you believe they will work for you? Because if you don't, they won't. Your intention won't be genuine, and your focus will be diluted by doubt.

The good news is, there are *many* reasons to believe that energy is real and that these practices will work for you, and you don't have to take my word for it. For thousands of years, practitioners from all walks of life have believed the universe is malleable. I can't wait for you to become one of them.

So, let's get into it!

CHAPTER 3

PUTTING ENERGY TO WORK

"All that you touch you change. All that you change changes you. The only lasting truth is change. God is change."

— OCTAVIA BUTLER, *PARABLE OF THE SOWER*

Scientists define energy as the ability to do work; with a few caveats, I think this definition fits our purposes well.

Work in this context means change, not productivity (the capitalist view of "work"). Change may mean speeding up or slowing down, heating or cooling, expanding or shrinking, pushing or pulling, or many other forms of transformation. I hope you are already seeing connections between this textbook way of describing energy and your own beautiful, complex human life.

There is no difference between the types of energy scientists postulate about (kinetic, potential, thermal, etc.) and the energy I teach you how to access in this book. The universe is teeming with energy; it connects us and every other being, known and unknown.

Human energy is not metaphorical. It is as real as electricity that lights your home and can be thought of within the same frameworks. In fact, the electricity in your body is largely responsible for your ability to hold this book and read these words.

My spiritual mentor, Dr. Kate Tomas, was the person who first encouraged me to think about my energy as a source of personal power. It wasn't an easy leap for me, but why would it be? We are conditioned to demand evidence of things unseen, even when the evidence is all around us.

"Energy is everything and everywhere, and it's not always invisible," Kate says. "Sometimes it's very visible. It can take multiple forms. It can take material form. It can take the form of emotion. It can take the form of anxiety and intuition. It's not a substance that you can point to necessarily, but it can become a substance. I think the best analogy is that we're fish and we're training ourselves to know that we're wet. It's very difficult initially to see because we live in it all the time. We're so used to it. We don't know anything different."

Depending on which journals you read, the universe is either made up of 70 percent energy or no energy. Team 70 Percent believes in an abundance of dark energy, a force that counteracts gravity and accelerates the expansion of the universe. Team Zero Percent believes in a perfect canceling out of positive energy (matter) by negative energy (gravity). Both models are useful.

If the universe is a closed circuit of energy and we are a part of it, that means anything we do will impact the balance. With practice and intention, we can learn to manipulate that impact and draw it into alignment with our desires.

If the universe is constantly expanding, that means the circuit is continuously growing more powerful, and our power grows along with it.

You're probably aware (perhaps painfully so) that our bodies contain their own energy systems. Think about the words we use to describe the way our systems and organs function. Our hearts *pump*. Our synapses *fire*. Our stomachs and intestines *metabolize*. There is change happening inside us all the time, and these internal energy systems influence how our bodies feel and function.

How we conceptualize the source, flow, and function of energy within our physical being depends on several factors, many of which are cultural. The emotions surrounding these concepts are fierce, in part because we humans are obsessed with how to explain this thing called *life*. Toss out a question like "When does life begin?" or "What happens to the energy in our bodies when we die?" and let the table-pounding commence.

The passion surrounding these concepts and questions makes sense because the mystery of our existence seems like the most important door we could ever unlock. For me, feeling like I've got it all figured out is the ultimate high. But I would argue that decoding the force that powers our universe is less important than believing in it and surrendering to its power. We can become so obsessed with figuring out the trick that we miss the true magic.

There's No Such Thing as "Good" or "Bad" Energy

When I first started using the word "energy" outside of physics class, I was a freshman in college, and it was almost always in a sentence like this: "I don't like hanging out with that guy. His energy is so *negative*."

My descriptive words for energy almost always fit into binary buckets: *good* or *bad*, *positive* or *negative*. I used them unthinkingly and without a lot of substance. For me, talking about energy was a shorthand way to explain how I felt around certain people.

How we feel around people is an important thing to pay attention to, especially for teenage girls living on their own for the first time. (I honestly can't believe that anyone is expected to leave home and lead a more-or-less adult life at age eighteen. I could barely pump my own gas, much less calculate compound interest or understand why 35-year-old men wanted to dance with me in clubs.)

But classifying energy as good or bad isn't a very nuanced way of thinking about *why* we like being around certain people over others. In fact, it's not an accurate way of thinking about energy at all.

For one thing, energy itself doesn't possess qualities like good or bad. It may behave as more or less "excited," meaning it vibrates at different frequencies, but energy itself is neutral; when put to work it produces results, and our human minds evaluate those results.

When we haven't thought about energy much, it's easy to evaluate a result as simply desirable or undesirable and to assume that the energy producing the result possesses the same quality. But as we become more skillful energy practitioners, we learn to harness neutral energy and manipulate it to help us achieve the results we desire.

This book, for example, will teach you the basics of how to direct your energy toward creating a fulfilling sober life. That's a complicated thing to do, and it doesn't happen by simply swapping out bad energy for good (if only it were that easy). Energy is a tool, and like any tool, it takes time to learn how to use it. Once you do, the world begins to feel like a very different place.

Let's go back to physics class. You probably learned that light is made up of photons, or particles that amount to bundles of electromagnetic energy. When these particles accelerate at a certain rate, the result is a visible light photon that can be seen by the human eye.

However, visible light is only a tiny fraction of the electromagnetic spectrum. Light is energy vibrating at a specific frequency, gathered and directed in a manner that allows the rods and cones in our eyes to register it. Visible light photons aren't better or worse than gamma-ray, infrared, or x-ray photons, but the way they behave together makes them useful to animals with eyes.[4]

The same concept applies to universal energy. It flows around and through us all the time, influencing our bodies, minds, and spirits. When we recognize the power we hold to manipulate that energy, the results are like turning on a proverbial light, illuminating a world of possibility we never knew existed.

How Does Our Energy Influence Our Emotions?

Eighteen-year-old me assumed that energy was measured or qualified by how it made you feel: good energy equals happiness, excitement, joy, clarity, and optimism, and bad energy causes sadness, anger, discomfort, confusion, and pessimism.

Energy *can* positively affect our emotions—but it's not as simple as turning up the flame on a burner and watching your feelings bubble with joy. A better analogy would be to think of energy work as your personal solar panel or wind turbine. With practice, you will be able to concentrate energy and use it to transform your life, the way a turbine captures power from the wind and transforms it into electricity.

Transforming wind energy into electricity can power a whole host of wonders that impact your emotions, from heating your home and powering life-saving medical equipment to blasting your favorite song or charging your vibrator.

Transforming psychic and universal energy into personal power can do the same thing on a similarly expansive scale. It allows us to change our lives in small ways that brighten our existence and draw our actions into alignment with our desires and values, yielding emotional and material benefits we never dreamed possible.

Will energy work make me happy?

Please hear this: I'm not saying that intention, meditation, aligned action, and integration are all you need to be happy (or sober). In fact, I want to poke at the idea that happiness should be our ultimate goal. *What is the energetic price of always striving to be positive and happy?*

Think about an experience that taught you something important or an event that you reference as a turning point in your life.

Now, project yourself back into the experience. I'm going to venture a guess that living through those moments (years, in some cases) wasn't exactly joyful. You may look back on it with gratitude or fondness; this is often the case when we accomplish a task that felt arduous at the time, like climbing a mountain. Or, maybe it's a painful memory of a challenging time, like the loss of a loved one or a relationship that wasn't right for you. Undoubtedly it sucked to live through but, ultimately, it may have opened an emotional or spiritual door. In both cases, we are better off for having these experiences even though they did not make us happy.

Here's another question: *What happens when we strive for happiness and fall short?*

For a long time, my brain operated on the assumption that the key to life was radiating positive energy and feeling only positive feelings. The unspoken subtext for this belief was that being positive would mean people would find me pleasant and enjoy being around me, which would result in my own happiness.

I now see this belief as a direct byproduct of being socialized as a woman: *My purpose and fulfillment come only from making other people feel good.*

It took years to untangle, but thankfully, I left this toxic idea behind (although I still see it occasionally loping after me in the rear-view mirror). Not only was it patently untrue that being relentlessly positive made me a people magnet, but it actually undermined the benefits I believed it would yield.

Don't get me wrong: There *are* tangible benefits to positivity, like faking it 'til you make it, training yourself to find gratitude, or letting go of negative thoughts that keep you stuck in the past. But setting the expectation that you should *always* feel happy, grateful, or loving is an almost surefire way to ensure that you don't.

Does this scenario sound familiar to you? You're scrolling through Instagram and see that someone you admire has posted a message about how much she loves herself despite not fitting a conventional set of beauty standards. In her post, she encourages her followers to buck socially constructed norms and to love themselves and their bodies.

But what if you are living with body dysmorphia or gender dysphoria or PMDD or just having a bad hair day? There are so many reasons why, at that moment, the well-intentioned invitation to love and accept yourself may feel impossible.

Intellectually, you may understand that you are entitled to positive and loving thoughts and feelings about your body. But what happens when those feelings remain elusive? What if the invitation to feel good about yourself makes you feel *worse*?

Even in my experience as a thin-ish white woman whose appearance checks many Euro-centric beauty boxes, looking in the mirror yields unpredictable emotions. And when I'm not feeling that great about what I see, that lack of affirmation bums me out on two levels.

One, I'm being an asshole to myself. Two, I'm painfully aware that I've succumbed to internalized misogyny, so I'm also being an asshole to women, girls, and people of all targeted genders. *Whomp whomp.*

For this reason, many voices in the gender justice and empowerment space advocate for body acceptance or neutrality as a goal rather than body positivity. Not that positivity isn't a fantastic goal, but it's aspirational. If we were playing The Legend of Zelda, body positivity would be Death Mountain. But many of us need to spend some time in The Lizard or even The Eagle before we'll make it there. Some of us stall out at The Dragon, and that's okay.

Energy work can be an enormously useful tool in the journey toward self-love. But there's a hell of a lot of unlearning that has to happen, and it takes time. Subscribing to "positivity or bust" can make it take longer.

Is energy the same as "vibrations"?

If you've spent any time hanging out in the personal development world, you've undoubtedly come across an idea referred to as *the law of attraction*. Abraham Hicks, Napoleon Hill, Louise Hay, and many others have made millions preaching the gospel of this universal "law."

In the simplest terms, the law of attraction states that we attract into our lives that which we think or focus our energy upon. By tuning our internal vibration to the frequency of what we want, we can manifest our greatest desires. Conversely, when we project negative thoughts and vibrations, we attract negative outcomes.

There's something incredibly seductive about the law of attraction. For one thing, it alters our perceptions of the barriers that stand between us and the life we want. This is a good thing. My training and experience in energy work support the belief that we have more power than we think we do to transform our lives. Energy—as we've discussed—is the ability to do work and create change. If we calibrate our energy to achieve the change we want, it is much more likely to happen.

But what troubles me (and many other teachers) about this approach to self-development is that it encourages us to causally trace our life outcomes *only* to the vibrations we omit—regardless of our identity, location, or life circumstances. The law of attraction does not account for the fact that not everyone's advantages and barriers are equal.

For example, many uncritical followers of this law believe that if they are successful, it is because they broadcast a more successful vibration. People who live in poverty do so because they "think poor." If law of attraction gurus ever acknowledge the realities of structural or systemic oppressions (racism, sexism, classism, ableism, homophobia, transphobia, etc.), it is usually unsubstantial and only in passing.

This way of conceptualizing energy is dangerous for a number of reasons. Most insidiously, it places the responsibility *and* the credit for any life outcome exclusively on the individual and their actions. Heredity, bigotry, or natural disasters interfering with your dreams? You're simply not thinking positively enough. Life beating you down? Raise that vibration, you loser!

The law of attraction also ignores the fact that humans are social animals whose development and evolutionary success are fundamentally tied to living in community. Sometimes, you'll hear a high-vibes evangelist talk about the abundance in the universe and how there is plenty for everyone. It sounds like they're preaching about a utopia where we all help each other, right?

Not in Law-of-Attraction Land. Here, believing in abundance is simply a vibration-raising tool. You believe in abundance so you can get more of whatever you want—for yourself. Everyone has access to this giant cosmic cash machine, so why should we make withdrawals for anyone else?

This is another reason the law of attraction is so popular: It validates the idea that we have no obligation to one another and absolves us of any responsibility to confront social or financial injustices.

Should we completely discard the law of attraction? As interpreted by Hicks, Hill, and Hay, I say yes. But let's not disadvantage ourselves by throwing all energy and manifestation work out with it. As Kate Tomas explains, once we embrace energy work that is empowering, communal, and liberatory, we realize that the law of attraction could never do what it claims to, anyway.

"How wonderful would it be that all the power in the whole world is just in your own hands?" she says. "The irony is: It *is*, but not as an individual."

> *Infinite capacity to change the world happens when we are in community. That's the truth of it. And the law of attraction is so harmful because its entire premise is that individualism is the route to success, to happiness, to peace. And the reality is community is the root of all of that. Individuality divides and separates us from the source of our power.*
>
> *When we focus on becoming sensitive to and mindful of our own energy centers, we suddenly understand how we are connected to everyone and everything. We're not trying to take control of our energy centers so that we can pull energy back and reserve it just for ourselves and focus exclusively on our entrepreneurial growth. No. We're connected. As soon as you become aware of true energy, you realize that you are not an individual. Individuality is a full lie. It's a complete fabrication. We are all everyone and everything. That is the nature of energy work.*

CHAPTER 4

WHAT IS BIG SOBER ENERGY?

"No solution can possibly exist while you're lost in the energy of a problem."

— MICHAEL A. SINGER

Look around you. Unless you're in a *very* remote area, everything you see started as a spark in someone's mind. The park bench you're sitting on. The book or device you're holding. The bulb that's lighting your room. Those things are physical manifestations of ideas—energy that coalesced in someone's brain and became tangible in the physical world.

Sometimes that thought is unintentional, as inspiration is for many artists. My favorite songwriter, Nick Cave (also in recovery), talks about sitting down to write because he has to; when inspiration strikes, the lyrics bypass his rational mind and pour out of him onto the page. He wrote *Push the Sky Away,* one of my most-played albums, in this manner.

But sometimes brain energy serves a deliberate purpose. An inventor, for example, may create multiple iterations of a widget before she successfully solves the problem that's been vexing her for years. (I, for one, am waiting for someone to invent a combination Snuggie- sleep-mask-headphone-neck-pillow so I can pack ONE THING and finally get some rest on airplanes.)

Inventing Your Sobriety

We can be like inventors. If we know we want to live a life that feels full and joyful without alcohol, we can begin focusing our brain energy on that vision. It might take a while, depending on the obstacles in our lives. We might not get it right on the first or second or third try. But if we remain curious and connected to our intention, we can invent our own sobriety.

If we *don't* know what we want (or we think we do but neglect to imagine it with any clarity), then our energy tends to leak out in random directions. We're shooting in the dark, hoping we'll hit the bullseye when all we're doing is wearing down our reserves.

When I was drinking, I ran my poor thoughts ragged, forcing them to chase a constantly moving target. A day in the life of my mind looked something like this:

> *"I really need to quit drinking. That's it; I'm done."*
>
> *"Actually, I just need to learn to stop after two or three. That should be easy. I don't want to be fully sober."*
>
> *"Do people talk about how drunk I get?"*
>
> *"I have a big weekend coming up. Fuck it. I deserve to have a good time."*
>
> *"I wonder if my thesis would be done by now if I didn't drink."*
>
> *"Who doesn't drink? Nobody, that's who. That is completely unrealistic."*
>
> *"I don't want to be some boring, moderate person. I love my wild self!"*
>
> *"I hate waking up every day wondering who I have to apologize to. This suuuuucks."*

I'm exhausted just reading over this tortured transcript. Now, imagine going through some version of that inner dialogue *every day*.

If you're reading this book, maybe you don't have to imagine it. Maybe this is your reality, and if that's the case, I'm truly sorry you are struggling. But in any case, it should be clear that these thoughts only led to anxiety, self-doubt, and paralysis. No wonder I kept drinking.

At an earlier point in my life, I would have paid someone a LOT of money to teach me to think the "right" thoughts, order them correctly, and Think Like a Sober Person.™ Unfortunately, no such recipe exists (although there are plenty of recovery gurus who will tell you it does).

It doesn't exist because sober people don't all think the same way or want the same things.

It doesn't exist because people with substance use disorder don't share one type of brain that changes predictably when fed the same diet of treatments, affirmations, advice, or beliefs.

And it doesn't exist because, to think like another person, you would have to *be* that person. You would cease to be you, and that would be a terrible loss to the world.

I don't have a recipe to give you, but guess what? You get a much cooler metaphor.

When you allow yourself to dream a big juicy dream about what you want your life to look like, when you can see it clearly in your mind's eye, and when you believe it's possible for you, those thoughts crystallize into your very own sobriety prism. When you project your energy toward the prism, its angles and shapes refract the energy based on *your* vision, *your* dream, and *your* desires for *your* life. The prism concentrates your energy and directs it, creating a cascade of colorful light, illuminating the path that leads you where you want to go.

The prism metaphor helps us learn to think like the version of ourselves who is already living our best sober life. I'm one of those people who believe there are multiple versions of reality happening at the same time. You don't have to believe that (obviously), but suspend your disbelief for a moment.

Do you know that old Gwyneth Paltrow movie *Sliding Doors*? There's a Sliding Doors version of you who doesn't drink and is kicking ass right now. You find her by learning to ask yourself, over and over again, "*What would Sliding Doors me do?*" You find her by making subtle micro-shifts that line up the pieces of your life like pins in a tumbler lock, opening the door to this new reality with a satisfying *click*. You find her by following the rainbow cast by your sobriety prism.

That's Big Sober Energy.

Plugging the Energy Leaks

If you aren't familiar with Bhante Gunaratana, it's my honor to introduce you. He's the author of *Mindfulness in Plain English* (among other books) and a philosopher whose writing I find myself returning to over and over and applying in almost every area of my life.

Gunaratana tells us that most humans categorize their experiences and emotions as either positive, negative, or neutral. We tend to hold tightly to the experiences we've labeled as positive. We chase after them and attempt to recreate them when they elude us. We dream about them and stake our happiness on them, casting unintentional spells by whispering to ourselves, "If only...."

This phenomenon is particularly acute for people with substance use disorder because our brains engage in selective memory when it comes to drinking and its consequences. Despite mountains of evidence to the contrary, our addicted minds hypnotize us into believing that drinking is a positive experience, thus intensifying the urgency of the chase.

Conversely, our brains do everything we can to avoid experiences and emotions labeled as negative. We fight them, deny them, and run from them. We're so afraid of bad things happening that we obsess about even the possibility and inadvertently create a state of anxiety or panic without any discernible cause.

And our neutral experiences and emotions—the ones that fill most moments in our days—get very little of our attention. We're too preoccupied with chasing the good stuff and resisting the bad.

Gravitating toward pleasure and away from pain may seem like a natural, even evolutionarily necessary, response to the gauntlet of life. But the problem with this way of living, Gunaratana points out, is that it separates us from the essence of our experience: *change*.

"Moment by moment life flows by, and it is never the same. Perpetual fluctuation is the essence of the perceptual universe," he says. "Open your eyes and the world pours in, blink and it is gone. People come into your life and go. Friends leave, relatives die. Your fortunes go up, and they go down. Sometimes you win, often you lose. It is incessant: change, change, change; no two moments ever the same."[5]

Bhante Gunaratana is a Theravada Buddhist monk; his writing on this subject reflects some of the fundamental tenets of Buddhist philosophy (which, like most spiritual traditions, includes multiple and diverse interpretations), particularly when it comes to the dangers of attachment. When we struggle against change rather than perceive it for what it is, Gunaratana warns that the result is "a perpetual treadmill race to nowhere, endlessly pounding after pleasure, endlessly fleeing from pain, and endlessly ignoring 90 percent of our experience. Then we wonder why life tastes so flat."[6]

Mindfulness in Plain English isn't a book about substance use disorder, but I don't think I've read a better description of substance use disorder than "endlessly pounding after pleasure, endlessly fleeing from pain."

And, bringing it back to energy, where does running the perpetual treadmill race get you? The amount of energy we spend chasing highs and attempting to keep our lives from swerving completely off the rails is energy we cannot direct toward growing our careers, relationships, passions, or bank accounts. It's not that those things might disappear altogether, but if you've ever looked back at the relationship or career or financial choices you made while drinking and asked yourself, "What was I thinking?" the answer is likely that you weren't.

If you're like me, thinking was usually replaced by defaulting to the least-objectionable option. Instead of charting an affirmative path, my energy was spent on getting drunk, or wondering if anyone noticed I was drunk, or trying to survive my hangover while sitting at a desk under fluorescent lights for eight hours (again).

Once we are no longer obsessing about drinking or using (or agonizing about the consequences), we have so much freed-up power to work with! The key is recognizing we have that power and being very intentional about how we protect and direct it.

Moving Away from the Cliff Edge

People in recovery get a lot of advice; unfortunately, some of the widely-accepted "truths" that underpin this advice urge us to use our energy in ways that can inhibit growth and change. They may facilitate sobriety, but—and I'm about to say something controversial here—sobriety should not be our singular goal. There is a camp out there that likes to say things like, "Your only job is not to [drink/use/pick up]." I am not in that camp.

Of course, focusing exclusively on not drinking or using is less destructive than drinking or using. And, while we're in early recovery (typically defined as six months to a year depending on who you ask), the conscious energy it takes not to [drink/use/pick up] may be all-consuming, because we're literally re-learning how to live in an unaltered state. But living this way forever continues to define your life in terms of its proximity to alcohol and drugs. Energetically, it keeps us stuck in what author Catherine Gray calls "cliff-edge mentality."

"Many in recovery believe that unless us recoverees eyeball the cliff edge, we could somehow somersault over at any time," she explains in her brilliant (and hilarious) book *Sunshine Warm Sober: Unexpected Sober Joy That Lasts*. "Of course, the edge exists. It would be foolish to pretend it doesn't. But to me, staring at it constantly would be like an open-heart surgeon consistently reminding themselves they could kill a patient at any second, or a tight-rope walker staring down instead of keeping their gaze level."[7]

Perpetually staring at the cliff edge takes a lot of energy; to be honest, the thought of living in this state of hyper-vigilance is part of what kept me from quitting drinking for years when I knew I needed to.

I'm already an anxious person who gets easily sucked into shame spirals. I didn't want to live in my boozy past, rehashing my (many) rock bottoms, and constantly reminding myself that I was different from other people (i.e., "They're allowed to drink and I'm not because they don't slide into belligerent blackouts after four glasses of wine, and I sometimes do").

Now that I'm sober, I also don't want to fear my future, always worrying that I'm one slip away from destroying the sober life I've worked so hard to achieve. This simultaneous past-and-future tripping feels to me like the opposite of probably the *most* widely accepted recovery advice (and with good reason): *Take it one day at a time.*

Fortunately, there are writers like Gray and Gunaratana who helped me see that—with a few years under my belt—it's safe for me to take my eyes off the cliff edge, trust myself again, and *live in the now.*

Your Recovery Garden

This chapter only has about 30 metaphors so far, which seems like far too few, so let's introduce another one: The Recovery Garden.

It goes like this. Think of your life as a garden bed. Drinking or using are weeds that have taken over.

At first, we know we need to put most of our energy into removing those weeds, and we do. It feels satisfying. The weeds are gone, and we can see the rich soil. We monitor it obsessively for new weeds. We want to protect it at all costs.

But if we only remove the weeds, eventually the soil we've worked so hard to clear starts to look like an empty dirt patch. Not very inspiring.

Over time, we get tired of staring at the dirt patch. The weeds start to pop back up, and we don't feel motivated to remove them. We don't feel satisfied by the empty garden. It isn't bringing us much joy.

BUT what if once we clear the bed, we begin to fill our garden with flowers and veggies that *do* bring us joy?

Every new flower and bud we grow fills us with its beauty and makes us feel proud.

They also take up space so the weeds can't grow nearly as tall. We still need to remove them, but they're much easier to pull when the garden is so full of vibrant colors, glossy leaves, and solidly anchored roots.

The mistake many of us make in recovery is focusing only on removing the THING that's ruining our lives, leaving us feeling empty.

But you are meant to grow and experience joy. You don't have to chase after pleasure anymore, but you also don't have to deny yourself. You can be, in the words of Amanda Eyre Ward and Jardine Libaire, a "sober lush" who still loves beauty and adventure and *life!* (Read about their book on this topic in Appendix B.)

The difference is now your experiences will be unfiltered, and they will be all the more precious because they are *real*.

The recovery garden is unpredictable. You never know what might pop up. It may get a little wild at times. But wildness, too, is gloriously real.

It's OK to be afraid of the realness. I suggest taking some deep breaths, sitting with it for a while, and watching what happens to your fear. Then repeat, and repeat, and repeat again.

(You may want to remind yourself of that when you get into Chapter 5!)

A Word About Energy Traditions and Cultural Appropriation

I mentioned earlier that there are many different approaches to energy work practiced around the world. Some focus on moving, healing, or releasing energy within and around the body. Some focus on connecting intentionally to universal energy. And some move between the two.

Similarly, there are many ways of naming and conceptualizing different forms of energy. These are usually culturally specific.

If you practice yoga, you may be familiar with the Sanskrit word prana, which is often used to mean breath but can also translate to life force or energy.[8]

In Greek, the word pneuma refers to one's breath or life or vital spirit.[9]

In Chinese medicine and culture, chi or qi is also commonly translated as a life force. A more nuanced understanding contextualizes this force as a function of fluctuating energetic relationships that impact balance and health.[10]

Ki (the root of the word reiki), translates from Japanese as "energy of everything" and is used as the root of many words and expressions.[11]

In Sufism, each person possesses a ruh, or an essential self, akin to a spirit or soul.[12]

The word loong in Tibet means mobility, referencing how energy moves through our organs and bodily systems as well as the movement of the mind.[13]

Mana, a concept important in Polynesian cultures, references energy derived from a supernatural nature. In Hawai'i, for example, some locations and beings are thought to have more mana than others.[14]

And nwyfre is a Welsh word that means vigor and is used by modern Druids to mean life force.[15]

These are only a few of many examples. I offer them to point out that the concepts of spiritual energy, collective energy, and energy work are only universal to a degree. The nuances and differences and specific spiritual origins matter, but this fact is often overlooked in modern spiritual teaching.

When a teacher engages in spiritual practices without properly training or acknowledging its origins, or worse, goes against the explicit wishes of the people who do practice the religion or philosophy, that teacher is guilty of cultural appropriation. This is compounded when the teacher is making money.

Cultural appropriation is rampant under capitalism. Many brands you are probably familiar with took their names directly from sacred ideas. For example, if you Google the word "prana," the first thing that comes up is a yoga clothing company. If you look up "mana," you will find websites selling energy drinks of the same name.

In spiritual communities, cultural appropriation takes many forms:

> Trading in spiritual ideas without referencing a specific tradition or source, even implying that the teacher themselves is the source.

> Divorcing the tradition from its unique cultural context or mixing ideas across cultural traditions without giving those traditions—or the people who practice them—the respect they deserve.

> Practicing rituals a teacher is unqualified to perform, thereby taking money away from people who have much deeper ties to the tradition in question.

A classic example of cultural appropriation is non-Native spiritual teachers using sage to "cleanse" their clients of malevolent spirits or negatively charged energy. I used to use sage casually in my own home, and I am so grateful to the Indigenous teachers who educated me about why this practice is harmful.

Sage is a sacred plant to Native Americans. Native people in what is now the United States are survivors of genocide. Generations of Indian children were forcibly removed from their homes and converted to Christianity, and many Indigenous adults were jailed simply for practicing their religion.

When white people use sage in generic "cleansing" rituals, they are essentially reinforcing the dynamic that white people can take whatever they want from Native people—even something sacred that Native people have fought and died for the right to practice.

Sage is also endangered due in large part to spiritual white people creating such demand for it. Its scarcity is yet another example of Native folks losing something sacred to them because white people decided they wanted it.

 I am saying all of this because I want to be clear that what I'm sharing with you in this book is partly derived from traditions outside my cultural or religious lineage. I want to be as transparent as possible about where these practices came from and how I came to learn them.

For example, I am not a Buddhist, but I have included some passages that were written by a Buddhist monk who offers his wisdom freely in the hopes that others will use it. I am not a Hindu, but I have included my modern, Western interpretation of a practice that references the concept of chakras, being clear that it is only one of many interpretations.

The things I am going to teach you about are not original to me, nor were they original to the teachers I've learned from over the years. In many cases, these practices have their origins in ancient or Indigenous traditions, and I have done my best to note where that is true. But most have evolved through time and space. They have become modern interpretations and should be understood as such. By writing about them in a recovery context, I have added another layer of interpretation.

I encourage you to research these traditions beyond what you will learn in this book. I have included a handful of primary sources from which some of these practices originated in Appendix B.

Support and read the work of people and communities that generously share their traditions. Respect their wishes when they do not wish to share them. Learn the difference between traditions that are open (meaning it is OK for people outside the religion to practice them) and those that are closed (practices restricted to only members of the religion).

Guarding against cultural appropriation is the right thing to do. It also makes a difference to our efficacy as practitioners. If energy is neither created nor destroyed, what happens when we behave in extractive ways? When we take without asking or giving back?

Simply put, if we belong to any dominant cultural identity groups, engaging in cultural appropriation will interfere with our energy work.

I say this as someone who has made many mistakes in this arena and will undoubtedly continue to do so. There is much to learn. I invite you to let go of any desire to do it perfectly. Dive into this work in the spirit of good intentions and deep listening. Extend care and respect to the incredible web of ancestral energy you will draw from and contribute to throughout your journey.

PART II

THE PRACTICES

MINDFUL ENERGY: NAVIGATING YOURSELF

Discovering your sober self is, I would argue, the most magical and rewarding aspect of recovery. After spending so many years avoiding your own eyes in the mirror, coming home to yourself can change everything—but it doesn't happen easily or all at once.

Knowing how to celebrate and care for ourselves while also holding ourselves accountable and figuring out how to be a person without alcohol is no small task. The practices in this section are designed to help you take small manageable steps toward establishing a strong and loving relationship with yourself. *This must be your primary and most important relationship!* Build a foundation of self-trust and compassion, and feel your power in recovery grow.

CHAPTER 5

HOW DO I FEEL?

"Emotions are celebrated and repressed, analyzed and medicated, adored and ignored—but rarely, if ever, are they honored."

— KARLA MCLAREN

My emotional life while boozing would have made an excellent example for a teacher explaining compound sentences to her English class.

> *I feel happy, but I could feel even happier if I drank.*
>
> *I feel sad, so I'd better drink.*
>
> *I feel bored, and you know what cures boredom? Drinking!*
>
> *I feel anxious at this party because I don't yet have a drink in my hand.*

Giving up that compound sentence life is not for the faint of heart. For me, it is the hardest part of being sober: feeling my feelings without immediately wanting to change them.

That urge hasn't disappeared. I still find myself trying to escape discomfort or enhance my mood via food, meditation, avoidance, sleeping, and binge-watching reality TV. I still fall into the trap of thinking I should or could feel different than I feel. I still find myself trying to secure my ticket to "not this" without bothering to explore what "this" actually is.

The urge may never leave me, but I also know it doesn't serve my higher self: the Sliding Door version of me who is living her (my) best and lushest sober life.

That version has accepted the fact that life is a water slide full of twists and turns. My first instinct might be to stiffen my body or flip myself over and attempt to scramble back up the slide. My Sliding Door self knows that to avoid painfully smacking against the side, I need to relax, go with the flow, and take the ride.

Sliding doors don't have keys, but if they did the key would be this: Get in the habit of asking yourself, "How do I feel?" and *not immediately doing anything about it.*

It sounds simple—and it is—but it's also a lifelong practice. For some of us, it goes against our first instinct, but it's worth it to pause and get curious. Honoring our emotions may be the single most transformative thing you can do for yourself as a person in recovery. Noticing without striving, observing without jumping into action, anchors us in the current moment and allows us to see things as they *are*, not as we wish them to be.

Asking ourselves how we feel also gives us incredible data to work with as we're trying to figure out how the fuck to be a person without alcohol to soften the emotional gauntlet of life. What does your antenna tell you about accepting a coffee invite from your nosy neighbor? What happens in your body when you attend a baby shower where everyone except you and the expectant mother is drunk? What chemicals does your brain release when you tell your boss *yes* or *no*?

We're not taught to pay attention to these signs and signals, but once we learn to do it, a whole new world opens up.

There are reasons other than substance use disorder that might cause a person to compartmentalize or resist fully engaging their feelings. For those of us who have experienced trauma, for example, numbing is a coping mechanism that may allow us to remain alive and functional. Deeply connecting with our feelings—and body sensations in particular—may not be safe or possible without additional support. Once that support is in place, however, not only can we find healing, we can find power. (Mindful movement also has tremendous benefits for trauma survivors who wish to explore their interior lives, as we'll discuss in Chapter 7.)

INTENTION

Intention and feelings may not seem like they belong together. Can we really *intend* to feel a certain way? And isn't that the opposite of honoring our emotions as they are?

Again, the idea here is not to transform feelings you don't want into feelings you want. The intention comes from noticing your feelings so you can become more informed and deliberate about how you support yourself emotionally.

For me, the act of observing my feelings yields powerful aggregate data and makes the waterslide of life a little less jarring. It shows me the value of minimizing my contact with people who sap my energy. It prompts me to schedule my writing time in the morning when I'm most creative. It reminds me to eat protein for breakfast so I can focus better during the day.

I can't control everything, but asking myself "how do I feel?" allows me to make the best decisions about things I can control.

Finding more ease also frees up some emotional bandwidth for intentionally stretching yourself and leaning into discomfort for the sake of growth—a much more difficult prospect when we're battling avoidable, low-grade discomfort all day every day.

Emotional embodiment is another method for marrying feelings with intention. While mindfulness teaches us to notice how our feelings show up in the body, many teachers of manifestation encourage their students to practice embodying how they *want* to feel. I think of this practice as visualization for the body.

The theory here is that when we give ourselves space to imagine the sensation of success (whatever that means to you), we enhance our ability to make choices that bring that feeling to pass. I love the idea of this practice but offer two caveats.

One, it is incredibly tempting to jump over the "how do I feel" step and go straight to "how do I want to feel." But manifestation isn't about creating the reality you want in that very instant. It is about deliberately manipulating your energy *over time* to assemble a future that aligns with your intentions.

You can't manifest the future you want if you are unwilling to sit with your emotions. Striving and straining are enemies of manifestation.

The second caveat is that I personally find this manifestation practice very difficult. I can visualize images and scenarios easily, but connecting to feelings takes a lot of effort. I still try because, intellectually, I see the value, and like most practices, it does get easier over time. But know if this one feels out of reach, you are not alone.

MEDITATION

Sitting for a daily meditation practice is the fastest and most effective way I know of to establish the habit of noticing your feelings.

For one thing, there's not much else to notice (other than your thoughts, which will do everything in their power to drag you away from your feelings).

For another, the repetition and regularity allow you to gauge how you feel from day to day to day. (The meditation app Insight Timer even has a "How are you feeling today?" feature that can help you track your emotional data points and the variables that may influence them.)

But the true magic here lies in the power of mindfulness, because once you get used to observing your mind during meditation, it becomes habitual. You will naturally start to observe your feelings and reactions throughout the day. You will develop the ability to connect to your meditative mind during moments of anxiety or uncertainty. These skills free you from the limits of your knee-jerk reactions and unveil infinite possibilities for how you can respond instead.

ALIGNED ACTION

When a strong emotion comes whipping around the corner and smacks you in the face, chances are you're not going to be in the headspace to engage in a complex thought or action. You need something that your brain can access quickly and easily in the midst of internal chaos. My favorite practice for this moment is a four-step process called RAIN.

RAIN

RAIN is a practice based in Buddhist philosophy and popularized by Michele McDonald, Tara Brach, and other modern mindfulness teachers. It's an acronym; everyone seems to agree on the *RAI* part, and there are several versions of *N* floating around. (I'll share my favorites with you, but no judgment if a different *N* floats your boat!)

1. R stands for *recognize* your feelings. It is the equivalent of asking yourself, "How do I feel?"

2. A stands for *accept* and *allow*. Let those feelings simply be without judging them or trying to change them.

3. I stands for *investigate*. This step invites you to be lovingly curious. What is this feeling telling you? How is it manifesting within your body? Is there something going on that might be exacerbating this feeling for you right now?

4. N stands for either *nurture* or *non-identification* (depending on who you talk to). Nurture reminds you to extend kindness and comfort to yourself in that moment. Non-identification invites you to recognize that you are not your feelings. Just because you might be feeling worthlessness, for example, does not mean you are worthless.

RAIN has been a lifesaver for me, particularly in situations where people around me are drinking heavily. These experiences no longer make me want to drink, but they sometimes make me uncomfortable and trigger feelings of disgust and resentment that I no longer "get" to participate in the debauchery. Even as my friend is slurring the same story at me for the third time and reminding me of why I DO NOT MISS DRINKING, I still feel a sense of loss.

I can *recognize* that I feel the loss of the life I once had and even grieve it to some extent.

I *accept* that these feelings are there and *allow* myself to sit with them in the moment.

When I *investigate* the circumstances surrounding these feelings, I realize that I know far more people who drink than who don't, and that I'm currently in a situation where that disparity is more obvious than usual.

Finally, I *nurture* myself by affirming that I have made a loving choice for myself, and practice *non-identification* by reminding myself that, even if I feel resentment in the moment, I'm not a resentful person.

RAIN allows me to quickly acknowledge how I feel in a given moment. It gives me the space to recognize that, even though the feeling may be unpleasant, it is part of a rainbow of authentic emotions that I *get* to feel now that I'm sober. And the feeling is a result of a complex decision that I make for myself every day out of bravery and love. Arriving at that realization almost always lifts my spirits.

INTEGRATION

Often, noticing how we feel and giving ourselves permission to feel it provides its own source of integration. Observing our emotions from a distance reminds us that they are temporary and takes the urgency down a notch or two. Once we are no longer being tossed about on the waves of our feelings, we can reflect and make meaning of them through talking, journaling, creating art, or saying words of affirmation to ourselves.

But if you do find yourself in a state of anxiety, overwhelm, or panic, you may notice physical responses that make it more difficult to find the distance between you and your emotions. Your adrenaline pumps, you get sweaty, and your gut starts to clench—all signs that you have activated your sympathetic nervous system. The "fight, flight, or freeze" instinct kicks in when we sense danger.

In these moments, staying present is much more difficult because the prefrontal cortex (rationality, forethought) is being overpowered by the amygdala (*I'm about to die, get me out of here!*).

When I find myself panicking, I put my hand on my heart. The warmth of my skin and the sensation of pressure against my body grounds and comforts me.

As weird as it sounds, I also force myself to hum or sing. These actions work because they help activate the parasympathetic nervous system, or the "rest and digest" activities in the body that allow us to recover after an intense or frightening experience.

Other practices that can help activate this system are deep breathing, taking a walk in nature, playing with a pet, gargling warm water, practicing tai chi or yoga, or getting a massage. Again, the goal of these actions is not to change your emotions, but to allow yourself to experience them without getting sucked into a spiral.

Activating the parasympathetic nervous system can also help restore your body's cortisol levels to normal, which is extremely important for avoiding stress-related symptoms and illnesses like high blood pressure, headaches, skin problems, and sleep disorders. When we "shake it off and move on" from a high-stress experience without integrating it, our cortisol levels can remain chronically elevated. I can't overemphasize how valuable it is for your body *and* your mental health to—at the very least—breathe and meditate after an acutely draining experience.

The last integration suggestion I want to make is to encourage you to befriend your brain.

Your brain is fucking amazing, but for those of us whose mental health puts us through the wringer, it can feel like an adversary. These embattled feelings are complicated by giant philosophical questions like, "Is the brain the same thing as the mind?" and "Where does the essence of self come from?" Regardless of what you think about the answers to those questions, learning a little bit of neuroscience can save you a lot of energy and self-loathing. It is worth your time.

When I was drinking, I had no understanding of where cravings came from. For over a decade, I labored under the belief that I drank too much because I was pathetic and weak, a loser with no willpower.

But did you know that, from a neuroscience perspective, *willpower doesn't exist*?

I learned this fact from a neuroscientist and addiction psychiatrist named Dr. Jud Brewer. If you want to learn more about the basics of how your brain works, neuroplasticity, and the reward system, I wholeheartedly recommend his book *The Craving Mind: From Cigarettes to Smartphones to Love — Why We Get Hooked and How We Can Break Bad Habits*. (Spoiler alert: He's a mindfulness geek, too!)

Dr. Jud was my first exposure to the concept of the reward cycle

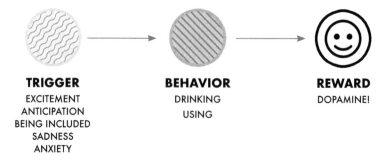

TRIGGER
EXCITEMENT
ANTICIPATION
BEING INCLUDED
SADNESS
ANXIETY

BEHAVIOR
DRINKING
USING

REWARD
DOPAMINE!

(sometimes known as the context-dependent memory cycle). The cycle has three stages: 1. trigger > 2. behavior > 3. reward.

- The trigger could be anything, really: sadness, celebration, the desire to fit in.

- The behavior is drinking (or smoking or any other compulsive behavior).

- The reward is the release of pleasurable brain chemicals that comes from engaging in the behavior.

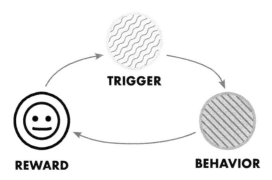

TRIGGER

REWARD **BEHAVIOR**

These three steps don't become a cycle until we repeat them. After experiencing them enough times (that number is different for everybody), people with alcohol use disorder begin to associate their triggers with the reward of an alcohol-induced dopamine rush. Once that association happens, it diminishes our ability to alter our behavior. The desire to drink starts to feel more urgent, eventually mimicking the fight-or-flight response. The urgency overpowers the parts of our brains responsible for engaging in long-term thinking or delayed gratification.

Not only that, but the reward we've been craving starts to shrink. Now, it takes more and more alcohol to appease the trigger and bring us base to baseline. Eventually, we're drinking to overcome the emotional deficits caused by drinking.

To put it more succinctly, we can't reliably resist or control our cravings just because we want to. Our brains will always want alcohol more.

The whole "willpower doesn't exist" thing would have been nice to know before I spent 10 years beating myself up for not having it. But once I did learn about the power of the brain's reward system, it was an absolute game-changer. That knowledge allowed me to forgive myself and put my energies toward recovery practices that work, like learning to tolerate my triggers and replacing my reactive behaviors.

Knowing that I had the power to intentionally change my brain reversed my beliefs about my capacity to become sober. It transformed my self-loathing into self-knowledge. It cracked open the door and let in enough light for me to finally see a way out.

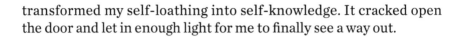 *For more on the relationship between mindfulness and the brain science of addiction, check out my article "Mindfulness Over Merlot" for Spirituality & Health at* **bigsoberenergy.com/ reader-bonuses.**

CHAPTER 6

SELF-COMPASSION V. SHAME

"Shame corrodes the very part of us that believes we are capable of change."

— BRENÉ BROWN

Writing a book about recovery is a bit of a mind fuck. Yes, you want to help people, and to accomplish this, people need to read your book. But do you actually want everyone to know the truth about all the gnarly, sketchy things you did before you got sober?

Cringe.

Luckily, I have some practice surviving this type of vulnerability. But it took a lot of baby steps to get to the point where I can share my story without immediately having to bury myself under a pile of blankets.

In 2020, I made the decision to "come out" publicly as a sober person on an episode of my podcast, *Feminist Hotdog*. That episode was a big deal for lots of reasons, not the least of which was that I got to interview Holly Whitaker. Holly is the pioneering founder of the recovery tech platform Tempest and a legend in the sober community. At the time, she was promoting the release of her groundbreaking book *Quit Like a Woman*.

Holly's episode was the first in a three-part series I produced on feminism and sobriety. As I worked on the series, it became obvious that I could not commit multiple episodes to this extremely complex topic and not be transparent about the fact that I had also left alcohol behind. That omission felt disingenuous, and recovery and disingenuousness don't mix for me.

There was just one problem. I hadn't had a direct conversation with anyone in my family about why I quit drinking.

It's not that I thought they would judge or reject me, exactly. My concern was more about worrying them and disappointing my parents. They were (and are) amazing parents; I didn't want them to think they had done anything to contribute to my substance use disorder. But I also didn't want them to hear I was sober (or about the cringe-worthy moments that led me to become sober) from a podcast.

The interview with Holly was recorded, the audio was edited, and the graphics were prepped. Three days before I planned to release the episode, I sat down and wrote a 4000-word blog post about my decades of drinking and how I finally got sober.

 To read the full post, visit **bigsoberenergy.com/reader-bonuses.**

Then, I conjured all my courage and sent it to everyone in my immediate family with this email:

> *Hello family,*
>
> *Happy New Year to all of you. I am writing today with some more personal stuff (not really news) to share.*
>
> *As I think you all know, I don't drink anymore. We haven't talked about it much, and I haven't been very forthcoming about why because I prefer to be perceived as someone who always makes great choices and is always in control—someone to be proud of. Anyway, despite having a mostly good and productive and healthy/ happy life, I was not always making great choices or in control when it came to alcohol, and I have decided to be honest about*

that on my podcast and blog. Before I share it with the world, I feel like it is important to share it with you, the people most important to me.

I am not an alcoholic, nor do I judge alcoholics. I am someone who managed a poor relationship with alcohol for a long time and have chosen to end that relationship. I hope my sharing this with you is not upsetting and that you are still proud of me.

Thank you for your support, and please know that I am open to talking about this if you want to. I no longer feel bad about it, and I am in a place in my life, personally and professionally, where being open about my experiences cannot hurt me.

Thanks for reading/listening if you choose to. [essay and episode attached]

With much love,
Adrienne

When I read back over this email now, I can feel the tension in my words, the desire to sound confident when, inside, I was crumbling with anxiety.

I would word it differently now, and leave out the part where I deliberately distanced myself from people who call themselves alcoholics. But I'm still proud of the version of myself that wrote this email with trembling hands. I especially love the part where I said, "Being open about my experiences cannot hurt me." That's a pretty boss thing to say!

But even though I felt a little like a boss, I also felt like a mess. Hitting *send* on that email sparked a rush of relief followed by an anxiety maelstrom. I knew telling my family about getting sober would spark questions, at least in their minds. It's pretty obvious that most people don't give up alcohol unless the consequences of drinking far outweigh the benefits. Was I prepared to answer questions about what those consequences had been for me?

The breadth of these consequences is hard to explain, even now. Some took the form of behaviors that made me so ashamed I wanted to crawl into a hole and die, including:

- Driving drunk
- Getting kicked out of bars
- Slapping people
- Hooking up with strangers
- Arguing for no reason
- Gaslighting friends when they tried to confront me about any of the above

The list goes on. I rode the Hot Mess Express for *many* years.

But the thing that truly put me over the edge was the exhaustion of living in fear of my own actions. By the end, I had zero trust in myself or in my ability to change my behavior. Recognizing the glaring misalignment within myself became my version of rock bottom. It might have been invisible to the rest of the world, but it tore at me nonetheless.

That wound had recently started to heal when I wrote the email to my family.

Shame is paralyzing. Sometimes, the only way to escape shame is to force yourself to reveal it to other people. Brené Brown's work on vulnerability explains this so beautifully. I hadn't yet read her books in January of 2020, and I didn't yet have her eloquence to help me put words to what I was feeling. But deep down, I knew: *My ability to change is directly related to my ability to extract myself from the shame spiral.*

I was not going to have the life I wanted unless I got as honest with my people as I had finally gotten with myself.

I refreshed my email about 40 times that day. It was agonizing. But, within a few days, I heard back from every member of my family. Their messages were full of love and affirmation that they were proud of me regardless of my drinking *and* because of my choice to stop.

It was one of the best weeks of my life.

You probably did a lot of things when you were drinking that you are not proud of. If you find yourself visiting the underground cavern of shame, I get it—truly. But you don't have to stay there. It's incredibly difficult to flourish and grow when you're living in a hole.

Shame keeps us caught in a circular mind game, always asking: Do I "deserve" to move on and heal? When do we know it is safe to forgive ourselves? How much penance is enough?

From where I stand, you not only deserve it, you are entitled to it. I might even go so far as to say *you owe it to yourself and to the world* to forgive yourself, crawl out of the cavern, and blow up the entrance, so there's no going back.

Staying miserable won't help anyone you've hurt. And holding on to self-loathing energy will only prevent you from sharing your gifts with other people and the world around you.

So, how do you let it go?

INTENTION

Your primary and most important relationship is with yourself. This is true for everybody, but for those of us with substance use disorder, the stakes are higher. Treating yourself as a friend and ally acts as a powerful accelerator to healing. When every part of you works together, the impossible becomes possible.

Making friends with yourself is easier to write about than to do, but YOU CAN DO IT! I would go so far as to say you must.

The first step is to recognize the importance of giving your relationship with yourself your full attention. Decide that being in love with yourself is what you want, and focus only on *that*. It might feel unnatural or even selfish, but without setting this intention and committing to it, your energy won't know where to go.

Once you decide, you'll start to notice when your subconscious serves you up garbage. Instead of accepting those negative beliefs as truth, you can instead choose to feed your mind messages that remind you of your greatness. You can become your own champion, your own cheerleader, your own best friend.

MEDITATION

If it's not your natural operating mode, cultivating trust and compassion for yourself requires you to change your thought patterns intentionally.

You may default to thinking that you are weak, worthless, or have no discipline.

You may blame yourself for your substance use disorder.

You may ruminate on things you said or did while intoxicated and allow those events to rule your feelings about yourself.

These memories and narratives are powerful, but they are not more powerful than your mind. Once you set your intention to change these patterns, you can cultivate the skills to recognize and overcome them.

First, recognize that thoughts born from trauma and regret present themselves differently than truths or messages that come from your authentic self.

Fear-based thoughts are usually accompanied by knots in your stomach and a prickly feeling of dread. This is the energy of danger.

Messages from your authentic self arrive with far less fanfare. They may take the form of a friendly voice speaking in your head or a sensation of deep knowing. True inspiration usually lands with a gentle, satisfying *thud*, like a square peg dropping seamlessly into the square hole it has been looking for.

This is the energy of confident neutrality.

In other words, the intensity of a thought or feeling doesn't necessarily correlate to how real or true it is. Fear responses are designed to alarm us and jolt us into action. This is handy when we're fleeing saber-tooth tigers, but it's less handy when our brains send us outsized signals about something embarrassing we did five years ago.

The more experience we have observing how our thoughts arrive, the more skillfully we can tell the difference between manufactured danger and true wisdom from within. We can learn to discern which thoughts are worth listening to and acting on and which ones we can safely release.

One of my favorite meditation techniques to cultivate this discernment is called Opening to Self.

In an Opening to Self meditation, you first practice vipassana or insight meditation, focusing only on your breath until your mind is relatively quiet. (This doesn't always happen for me; sometimes, my mind has a mind of its own.)

When practicing this meditation, I'll often visualize myself opening a door, entering a room in my mind, and sitting down in a chair. Then, I ask myself: *What do I need to know?*

And then I listen.

Sometimes nothing happens. Sometimes messages appear in the form of a color or a sensation or a song. But every once in a while, I get a full-on message from my higher self. Some examples of messages I have heard are:

> *You don't need to lecture him. Just love him.*
> (In reference to my husband, who finds himself on the receiving end of far too many "helpful suggestions.")
>
> *Your life is better when it's filled with music.*
> (A nudge reminding me of how much more vibrant I feel when surrounded by sound vibrations.)
>
> *You should start a podcast and call it Feminist Hotdog.*
> (The inspiration for my first adventure in Audioland.)

Cool, right?

Even if you don't receive fully-formed messages, simply meditating regularly will help you discern your guilty or anxious thoughts from your more "skillful" thoughts, as Bhante Gunaratana calls them. The more quickly you can learn to identify thoughts that drain and misdirect your energy, the more easily you can brush them off before they latch on and burrow into your brain.

ALIGNED ACTION

Do you remember returning to school after the summer break between middle and high school? I do. In particular, I remember becoming obsessed with my formerly repellent lab partner who, in a scant three months, had transformed from a baby giraffe into a Luke Perry lookalike. (I'm dating myself, but Luke Perry's beauty transcends time and space. RIP, Luke.)

My relationship with affirmations is a lot like the 180 sparked by my lab partner's summer growth spurt. I didn't start out merely skeptical of affirmations; I thought they were pathetic. Influenced in no small part by Stuart Smalley (again, young folks may need to look that one up), I believed that only losers would waste time trying to pump themselves up while staring into their own eyes in a mirror.

To be fair, I had also believed sobriety was for losers, and that attitude hadn't worked out so well for me. So, when someone I respected suggested that I *try* affirmations before talking shit about them, I did. And I went from scoffing at the idea to becoming a devoted practitioner within a few short weeks.

No matter how awkward they seem, the bottom line is affirmations *work*. Science backs this up. In a 2016 study called "Self-affirmation activates brain systems associated with self-related processing and reward and is reinforced by future orientation," the authors state:

> *Affirmations can decrease stress, increase well-being, improve academic performance and make people more open to behavior change…. Self-affirmations are acts that affirm one's self-worth, often by having individuals reflect on core values, which may*

give individuals a broader view of the self. This in turn can allow individuals to move beyond specific threats to self-integrity or self-competence.[16]

When it comes to rewriting the subconscious narratives that influence our energy, affirmations are *the* most accessible tool I have found. You can use them anytime, anywhere, any way you want.

Your affirmations don't have to capture the greatest accomplishment or change you hope to make in your life, but rather something you would like your subconscious to help you either create or overcome.

When you're getting started, choosing from a pre-written set of affirmations can take the pressure off and allow you to begin experiencing the benefits without having to complete an assignment first. I have provided you with a few example sets, and Google offers a rich treasure trove of options.

But the most powerful affirmations are the ones you write yourself because they reflect your specific needs and circumstances. As Kate Tomas once told me, saying affirmations written by someone else is like wearing a shirt off the rack versus one tailor-made for you.

HOW TO WRITE AN AFFIRMATION

Step 1: Think about a realistic shift you want to achieve right now.
It's okay to dream big, but try not to pick something so outlandish that your mind will automatically reject it. For example, don't try to "affirm" your way to a million-dollar deposit in your bank account tomorrow; it doesn't work that way. (I wish it did.) If shifting money energy is your goal, a more realistic approach could be affirming that you are worthy of stability and success.

Step 2: Write an affirmative statement about that shift in the present tense.
Articulate the shift as if it has already happened. Using the example above, that statement could be something subtle like, "Every day, I

take steps to grow my wealth and secure my financial future." Or, take a simpler, more poetic approach, like, "I am magnetic to money."

Step 3: Say your affirmation at least three times in a row.

I was taught to say affirmations three times each, three times a day. The number three is key. The first time you say it, you won't believe it. The second time, your brain starts warming to the idea. By the third time, it really gets in there.

I rarely succeed at the three times a day part, to be honest. Doing it at all is more important than doing it perfectly. I am religious about saying affirmations in the morning, because that's what works for me. I encourage you to use your creativity to find what works for you. However you can regularly and repeatedly get the idea into your brain will be the most effective.

Some of my students record themselves saying affirmations and listen to them in the car.

Some write them on Post-Its and stick them strategically around their homes.

Some create sigils or glyphs by artistically combining the first letters of the words in their affirmations.

Some practice Emotional Freedom Technique (EFT) by tapping on different energy points on the body as they either say or listen to affirmations to amplify their effectiveness. (You'll learn more about EFT in Chapter 7.)

Here's an EFT affirmation script I wrote for people in recovery from substance use disorder who struggle to trust and forgive themselves.

1. Crown of the head: *Even though I hurt myself and others while I was drinking/using, I completely love and accept myself.*
2. Inside of the eyebrows (two hands, either side of the bridge of your nose): *I accept that I did the best I could with what I had at the time.*

3. Outside of the eyebrows (two hands, next to your temples): *I take full responsibility for my actions, even the ones I am not proud of.*

4. Under the eye (two hands): *I forgive myself for the things I said and did while I was under the influence.*

5. Upper lip (one hand, under your nose): *I am grateful for the people who helped me find this new pathway, even if they are no longer in my life.*

6. Chin crease (one hand, under your lower lip): *I release the need to redeem myself in the eyes of others.*

7. Chest (two hands, under your collarbones): *It is not necessary for other people to forgive me for me to forgive myself.*

8. Solar plexus (one or two hands, where your rib cage comes together): *I am inherently valuable and worthy of love.*

9. Underarms (one or two hands, reach across your body, and tap where your bra strap would be if you were wearing a bra): *I completely love and accept every version and piece of myself.*

10. Wrists (tap your wrists together): *I embrace my power to make choices that align with my values.*

11. Back of the hand (below where the ring and pinky fingers meet): *I am ready to heal the parts of myself that are still suffering.*

12. Side of the hand (below your pinky joint): *I send healing energy to every version and piece of myself, especially the ones I have been ashamed of in the past.*

13. Healing and loving myself is the greatest gift I can offer. (crown)

14. I attract people who see my worth and support my healing. (inner eyebrow)

15. I release all feelings of shame, guilt, and regret related to my actions while I was drinking. (outer eyebrow)

16. The more compassion I find for myself, the more power I have to show up authentically in the world. (under eye)

17. My value and entitlement to love are not determined by how other people feel about me. (upper lip)

18. I am grateful for the lessons I have learned. (chin crease)

19. I am confident in my ability to live in alignment with my values and purpose. (chest)

20. Every day, I take steps to build trust with myself. (solar plexus)

21. I forgive myself. (underarms)

22. I accept myself. (wrists)

23. I respect myself. (back of hand)

24. I love myself. (side of hand)

Tap on your body while you say or listen to these affirmations every day for two weeks, and watch the magic happen.

 To hear an audio version of this tapping script, visit **bigsober-energy.com/reader-bonuses.**

INTEGRATION

None of us can control how other people feel about us or whether they will ever forgive us for how we treated them while we were drinking or using. This can be hard to accept, but accept it we must if we ever wish to reclaim our energy from the toxic vortex of shame.

It is not necessary to obtain forgiveness from other people in order to forgive yourself. Please read that sentence carefully at least three times. Commit it to memory.

However, if you are struggling to move past memories of that hurt you've caused, apologizing is an avenue that's open to you.

Not to trivialize the art of apologizing, but it helps to have a formula. Without one, it's easy to get flustered and miss important pieces or misspeak altogether. I use the same three-part formula for apologies as I use to write thank-you notes. (Thank-you note etiquette was drilled into me as a child, so I can access it easily under stress.)

First, name the gift/grievance:

Thank You Note	Apology
Thank you for the beautiful Garfield stationery set!	*I'm sorry I borrowed $600 from you and never paid it back.*

Second, demonstrate that you understood the significance of the gift/grievance.

Thank You Note	Apology
It was so sweet of you to pick my favorite character. I love it!	*I know I violated your trust and put you in a bad spot financially.*

And, third, make a reference to how you will use the gift/grievance in your life going forward.

Thank You Note	Apology
I look forward to taking it to camp this summer so I can keep in touch with all my friends. Look for a letter from me!	*Knowing I hurt you has pushed me to start living within my means and stop borrowing money. I'd like to pay you back with interest. I'm really sorry.*

Then, STOP TALKING. The most important part of any apology is resisting the urge to excuse or over-explain your behavior. Own it, say you're sorry, name how you make amends and do better, and let that be it.

Remember: You can't make anyone forgive you, and forgiveness is not a prerequisite for your healing.

Before embarking on *any* apology to anyone for any reason, prepare yourself for the harsh reality that the person may (justifiably) refuse your apology or even unload their anger and resentment onto you. This might influence your decision to apologize in writing, via voice memo, or in person.

Regardless of the platform, the energy protection practices you will learn in Chapter 10 are non-negotiable before you make any apology.

Protecting your energy means holding no expectations about the outcome. Surrender that to the universe. Reflect on the experience of apologizing—whether it goes well or you get a cold, angry response—and put it behind you. To do otherwise is to risk sliding back into the shame cavern.

You can also apologize to yourself. Drinking and using in excess may have been an entirely understandable choice when you were making it, but it also hurt you. Knowing that you hurt yourself over and over can be the cause of subconscious resistance to change and growth.

Consider creating a ritual during which you write an apology to yourself and send it in a scheduled email at least a month out. Reading your own words when you don't remember writing them is a profound and powerful experience, so schedule it for a day when you anticipate having some head- and heart-space to spare. Trust me—you may need a minute.

I write and schedule emails to myself several times a year. Sometimes, I issue myself an apology, and sometimes, I send myself messages of encouragement or congratulations.

Each message reminds me of the day I received those emails of support from my family.

Each one fills me and my day with a deep sense of gratitude.

Each one connects me more deeply to my best self and reminds me that I am worth loving and protecting.

CHAPTER 7

BODY AND SOUL

"In order to change, people need to become aware of their sensations and the way that their bodies interact with the world around them. Physical self-awareness is the first step in releasing the tyranny of the past."

— BESSEL VAN DER KOLK

If you mapped my drinking over the years I was really going for it, the result would look like the graph on the next page.

The second big spike you see in the chart began in the summer of 2004. Thinking about this period still brings back the taste of Mike's Hard Lemonade mixed with bourbon, cigarettes, and cocaine. It's blurry. My weight plummeted. I was too high or hungover to eat most of the time. I threw up almost every morning. When I could choke it down, I lived on ibuprofen and coffee.

If you had asked me back then, I likely would have insisted I was having the best summer ever—that I was *thriving*. In reality, life as I knew it was ending, and I wasn't handling it well.

The reasons weren't all bad, but they were stressful. My nine-year relationship was coming to a slow, painful end. My best drinking buddy moved away. I co-founded a roller derby league, which required juggling the wants and needs of 90 highly opinionated women. I started graduate school and found I was older and had been away from the demands of academia much longer than almost all my classmates.

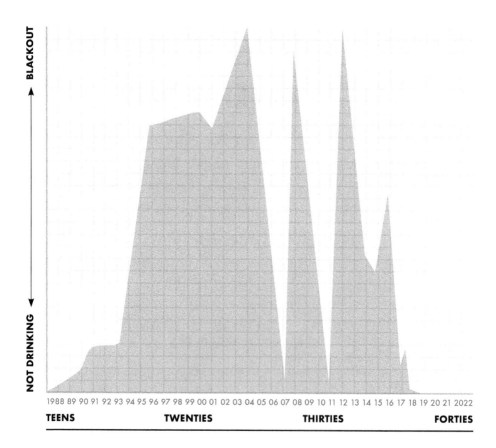

BLACKOUT

NOT DRINKING

1988 89 90 91 92 93 94 95 96 97 98 99 00 01 02 03 04 05 06 07 08 09 10 11 12 13 14 15 16 17 18 19 20 21 2022

TEENS   **TWENTIES**   **THIRTIES**   **FORTIES**

This moment could have been an invitation to settle into my 30-year-old self, and find a routine that supported days of immersive research, writing, and strolling amongst the university's lush trees and stately buildings (a fantasy life I had long romanticized).

But that's not what happened.

Instead, I started running with a wild (and, in many ways, wonderful) set of characters who took every opportunity to explore the limits of sleeplessness. I also moved in with a dancer from a local club who smoked meth daily and was having a dramatic affair with a famous (and married) artist/professor. As an individual, I had (and have) zero judgment about her choices. But as a living situation, chaos ruled our days.

My memories of this time are like a montage from a bachelor-ette-party movie, except my movie never ended. It's shocking to me that I didn't seriously hurt myself during this time, because my rational mind and my body were completely estranged from one another. I simply did not care what I drank, popped, smoked, or snorted. In my mind, I was living a glamorous double life of intellectual rigor by day and Dionysian excess by night. But in reality, I was assaulting my brain, lungs, and liver with punishing amounts of toxic substances, all while telling myself I was special because I had the guts to choose a lifestyle other people only experienced through films.

As you can see from the graph, the Hot Mess Express finally slowed down. Although hardly the picture of health, I eventually started sleeping and holding down food. But those spike months are notable to me, not just because of how extreme my behavior was, but because I barely allowed myself to think about them after I got sober. I simply could not come to terms with what I had done to my body. If I allowed myself to sit with my memories, to replay both the nights *and* the mornings after in my head, it looked less like a party and more like watching a stranger attempting to destroy herself.

I felt like my body was the scene of a crime.

Coming back from such profound and prolonged self-abuse and dis-connectedness was a slow and deliberate process for me. I wish I had had someone to tell me how to take my own hand and walk back toward some semblance of care and regard for my physical being.

I also wish I had known what readers of Bessel van der Kolk's work know: The body keeps the score. In other words, it manifests our trauma and pain in ways we may not recognize as trauma and pain. Without finding the places where pain has burrowed into our muscles, bones, and organs, we have a much more difficult time coaxing it free.

This was all news to me at the time. Despite my feminist leanings, "healthy = thin" was the paradigm I defaulted to, so that's the direction my feet were pointed when I first set out to sober up and repair the damage I had done to my body.

First, I ordered an elaborate "cleanse" that involved dozens of daily supplements and horrible-tasting powders. My weight was already low, so depriving myself of even more calories left me light-headed and unable to focus. After that, I adopted a restrictive diet and signed up for weight-lifting and cardio classes at the university, which meant that, including the roller derby practices, I was working out about 20 hours a week.

But the thing that made me feel the most virtuous was white-knuckling my way through my first three-month stint without alcohol.

"Look at me!" I thought smugly to myself. "Who goes from black-out drunk to star athlete in just a few weeks? I'm never going back to that unhealthy lifestyle."

But, again, that's not what happened.

Because you'll notice some key ingredients are missing from my transformation story: Therapy. Reflection. Research. Mindfulness. Connecting with other people who were making similar changes. *Making friends with my body.*

No healing had occurred. I had simply gone from pumping myself full of drugs to punishing myself with hyper-controlled eating and extreme levels of exercise. And I relied entirely on willpower—the patron saint of the quick-fix seeker—to do it.

The body does, indeed, keep the score. In my case, the score arrived packaged as a series of excruciating back and neck injuries. Getting to and from campus became a painful ordeal. My roller derby career effectively ended. And I started drinking again.

Let's travel to the end of the timeline. As you know from reading my story, it was a conversation with my body—a real one, not a lecture or a screaming match—that led to my finally getting sober for good. This time, I knew how to listen because I had been meditating. And, somehow (probably also through meditation), I knew instinctively I couldn't "fix" what was wrong with me by manipulating my diet or adding more cardio to my exercise routine.

Any course of action predicated on the notion that there was something wrong with me would inevitably fail and launch me right back into the cycle of punishment I had been living in for years.

Humans are not machines that can be fixed. If we think of ourselves as such, we'll inevitably end up disappointed because we can't achieve the impossible. Aiming for "fixed" is a set-up for failure.

Around the time I gave up trying to fix myself, I had the privilege of becoming a dedicated student and teacher of yin yoga, an asana practice in which you hold a series of static postures for long periods of time (up to ten minutes). The benefits are numerous, including greater flexibility, circulation, joint health, and stimulation of the body's energy centers.

Yin yoga is practiced under this name mostly in North America and Europe, where it was popularized by two teachers named Paul Grilley and Sarah Powers.

The origins of yin are debated, but I feel safe to say it is a modern interpretation of an ancient asana practice. Grilley was inspired by Taoist yoga,[17] a form of yoga popularized by martial artists. Other teachers trace yin's origins back to the *Hatha Yoga Pradipika*, a 15th-century text focused on preparing students' bodies for the rigors of extended meditation practices.[18]

However this approach to yoga found its way to the studio where I taught in Montgomery, Alabama, I'm grateful. My love of yin opened up an interior room where my body and I finally sat down and made peace with each other.

Being still with my thoughts and my breath while also being slightly uncomfortable for a long period of time wasn't something I looked forward to. Any new activity feels awkward or foreign at first, but this one carried an extra layer of "don't wanna" because it basically created a radio station for the voices in my head. But it also offered me an opportunity to examine those voices closely and recognize that many of them weren't actually me. And once the imposters revealed themselves, it became easier and easier to turn down the volume or tune them out altogether.

Being still is hard. Even though no strenuous effort is being exerted, having nothing to do but breathe and observe your mind and body often feels more taxing than pounding out miles on a treadmill. But yin is where I learned to use my breath to relax in places I didn't know I was holding tension. It's where I learned to speak kindly and encouragingly to myself. It's where I truly learned to meditate. And it's where I began to integrate my mind and body for the first time since I was a child.

INTENTION

I'll say it again: Coming back from fighting a long-term battle with the body is a slow and deliberate process. The intention I teach and recommend to anyone making a recovery transition is to embrace that deliberate energy. Move in service of your spirit, not your impulse to fix yourself.

Not everyone has access to gyms or time, as I did, to take formal yoga classes. Single moms and people who have three jobs will rightfully roll their eyes at the suggestion to "slow down." So, part of what I hope to inspire with this intention is finding micro-moments of slowness and movement wherever we can access them. Over the course of days, weeks, and months, those little moments can move internal mountains.

Many doctors, therapists, and other well-intentioned treatment providers suggest that sobriety-seekers add movement into their routines to boost endorphins and reduce stress. On the surface, there's nothing wrong with this advice. Unfortunately, because we live in a society that's not only obsessed with whiteness and wealthiness but also thinness and able-bodiedness, the message is often marinated in ableism, racism, classism, and diet culture.

As doctors and therapists come to know the work of Bessel van der Kolk and other trauma-informed researchers, I hope the recommendations to exercise will become less about "fitness" and more about equanimity. In our most vulnerable moments, we need movement practices that invite us to connect with ourselves *gently* and focus on breathing that matches a body at ease rather than a body under stress.

When it comes to movement, be the tortoise, not the hare.

Burning up the Stairmaster or pumping out chest presses may help you, too. If that's the case, by all means, go for it. But don't be afraid to dial down the intensity, listen, and give yourself space to explore a non-combative (or at least less-combative) relationship with your body.

You'll likely hear a voice in your head that says any exercise that's not burning calories isn't worth it. That's the voice of diet culture masquerading as you. But it's not you. If that happens, tell the voice, "I'm listening to my body right now, not you." Say it out loud!

If eating disorders, body dysmorphia, physical trauma, or any form of what Sonya Renee Taylor refers to as Body Terrorism[19] are part of your story (and I would be shocked if they were not), I want you to approach this slowing down with an open mind *and* a deep sense of compassion for yourself. Being still and slow might be intensely activating for you. You may find that your negative self-talk gets so loud it becomes unbearable.

If this happens, don't force yourself to push past it or gut it out. You may do better in a group or therapeutic setting or with a different movement modality or simply practicing for a much shorter time period. But keep listening to yourself and experimenting. There is no failure. Finding what feels good and liberatory for *your* body is the goal.

MEDITATION

Walking meditation is an ancient practice with roots in Mahayana and Theravada Buddhism. I was introduced to this meditation during my teacher training—and we were not friends. Annoyingly, I knew from my yin experience that the resistance I felt about walking meditation was an indication of my need for it. And so I walked. Slowly. Grudgingly.

Walking meditation or kinhin invites you to put one foot in front of the other in slow motion. (I always aim for the slowest I can move without falling over.) The idea is to feel and focus on every component of an activity many of us do every day but hardly ever think about.

Similar to examining the breath in vipassana, walking meditation asks the practitioner to examine the sensations involved in each stage of a step: lifting your heel, then your toe, moving your foot in front of the other foot, putting it down heel first, then flattening the first foot as you lift the second foot and doing it all again for about 10 to 15 paces.

If walking isn't accessible for any reason, you can do this meditation by creating a stepping motion on the floor from a sitting position. If your legs or feet don't move in that way, I suggest raising or lowering your arms, shoulders, or eyebrows. Whichever version you practice, the idea is the same: micromovements paired with deep, mindful observation.

Walking and other mindful movement meditations build body connection and awareness while explicitly discouraging judgment. Some people love it. People like me generally don't, at least at first. But despite my lack of enthusiasm, I sometimes find myself doing walking meditation almost without deciding to. That type of involuntary action used to happen to me with drinking. This is much, much cooler.

ALIGNED ACTION

At some point in your wellness journey, you may have come across practices described as *somatic*. Definitions vary, but I think of somatic work as anything that focuses on sensations inside our bodies rather than on the functional movements made outside. It's not an activity like tennis or squats, but rather, as somatic educator Elaine Colandrea[20] describes, an invitation to "move from inner sensation, curiosity, and pleasure, which brings us to an inner state of beauty, wholeness, and wonder."

There are many somatic practices out there. These are a few of my favorites. I hope they inspire you to keep exploring or even invent your own.

Self Massage

If you're like me, the only time you think about getting a massage is when you feel stiff or sore. But massage doesn't have to be reserved as a treatment for injury. There are lots of benefits to massaging our own bodies, but not a lot of encouragement to do it. Why? And why might even thinking about massaging yourself feel weird?

When I first heard about self-massage, it was in the context of "use a tennis ball to mimic that thing your massage therapist does with her elbow." It was about releasing the knots in my back, not feeling more connected to my body. And, yes, there are lots of therapeutic things we can do to release tension in our necks, etc. But what about massage for the sake of feeling your own skin? Making yourself tingle? Even rubbing in a little oil so you feel all soft and glowy?

Why do we have hang-ups about massaging ourselves?

My theory is that being sensual with ourselves in any way *still* carries a stigma for people raised as women. And for most people raised as men, self-massage would be acceptable only as an after-workout activity, not an act of self-love or self-care.

Basically, to avoid ever being labeled depraved (women) or feminized (men), we can only touch ourselves to stay clean and each other to have sex. Touching yourself for pleasure is a no-no.

When you see it spelled out in black and white, the whole idea that touching our own bodies should be any kind of taboo looks pretty dumb. But we absorb a lot of dumb things into our subconscious that require unlearning. This is one of them.

So, with that out of the way...

IT IS OKAY TO TOUCH YOUR BODY. Get yourself off. Stick sex toys wherever you want (just make sure they are clean). Pat yourself on the back. Hug yourself. Ritually cleanse your feet. Run your fingers through your hair. Squeeze your fat. Tickle your ribs. Rub the soles of your feet together. Drink juice out of your belly button with a long straw.

If nothing else, get some nice oil and rub it on the parts of you that you avoid looking at in the mirror. Your thighs are the Queen of Sheba. Your ass is Aphrodite. Your stretch marks are veins of gold, crisscrossing the world's most luscious landscape. Treat them like goddesses. Tell them you love them. Maybe even infuse the oil with self-loving energy before you begin. Make it magic. You are magic. Treat yourself as such.

If connecting with your body feels difficult, you are not alone, and there is nothing wrong with you. One of my favorite resources for building toward a more loving relationship with our physical selves is *The Body Is Not an Apology* by Sonya Renee Taylor and the accompanying workbook *Your Body Is Not an Apology*. I require my students to buy both of these books, and I return to them regularly whenever I notice myself looking away from my reflection in the mirror.

Utkata Konasana or Goddess Pose

Traditionally, yoga is taught and practiced as a sequence of postures that build on one another. I almost never suggest doing a single posture in isolation—unless it's one of the two I'm about to describe.

Several years ago, there was a TED Talk going around by a researcher named Amy Cuddy. Her work on the psychological impact of posture led her to theorize that when we stand in ways that take up space, we look more powerful and experience hormonal changes that cause us to feel more assertive.

In the classic power pose, you stand with your legs slightly wider than hip distance, chest open, arms akimbo, fists on hips, head held high. But I'll do you one better, or rather, the ancient Vedic practitioners of India will.

Utkata konasana, or goddess, is the ultimate power pose. To practice it, step your feet wide, toes turned out. Raise your arms over your head, then bend your knees into a squat, keeping them aligned with your feet. As you lower, bend your elbows to create "goal-post arms." Keep your chest open and your pelvic floor engaged. Spread your fingertips wide. If squatting is not accessible, you can practice with your arms and hands.

I like to raise and lower myself in and out of goddess pose a few times and sync the movement with my breath: inhale to stand, exhale to squat. The feeling of taking up space, fully engaging my body, and forcefully expelling my breath absolutely pumps me up and makes me feel strong. It makes me proud of the parts of me that I sometimes worry are "too big." It allows me to embrace my inner bad bitch.

Viparita Karani or Legs Up the Wall

You hear a lot in yoga circles about how *uh-ma-zing* inversions are for your body and mind. But many inversions are not accessible to people who aren't regular yoga practitioners. Even Adho Mukha Svanasana (downward facing dog) can be challenging for people who don't have a lot of upper body strength and impossible for many people with limited leg mobility.

My favorite inversion is Viparita Karani (often referred to as legs up the wall). It's not universally accessible, but it's available to people on a much wider spectrum of mobility than most other yoga poses that position your feet or chest above your head.

To practice Viparita Karani, sit on the floor and scoot your hips up next to a wall. If you want to elevate your hips, you can sit on a pillow; otherwise, keep your seat on the floor and extend your legs long. Then, reach your hands behind you, and either use your arms to rotate yourself or ask someone to help you rotate your body so that your back and head are on the floor. Your spine will be perpendicular to the wall, your seat pressed against the wall, and your legs either extending straight up the wall or bent—whichever feels the most relaxing and natural for you.

From a physical perspective, Viparita Karani increases circulation and helps release tension in your lower back—both good things. But I'm mostly a fan of the psychological benefits of this pose. Being held by both the floor and the wall makes me feel extremely supported. I also enjoy looking at my room from a totally different point of view. And I can shift my legs around to make different shapes, which helps me feel connected to my body in a way that feels fun and lighthearted.

Over time, practicing Viparita Karani and Utkata Konasana when you need comfort or strength will help your mind associate the physical practice with these feelings. The pose becomes a container within which you can connect with yourself. I even found that after having shoulder surgery that prevented me from practicing yoga for weeks, I could do these poses in my mind and feel the benefits. We can use our bodies to access our minds—and vice versa.

INTEGRATION

Your relationship with your body can be a source of anxiety and an instrument to measure your emotional state. It can also be a means to integrate stress, triggers, and cravings.

EFT or Tapping

I mentioned Emotional Freedom Technique (sometimes called Energy Freedom Technique, EFT, or tapping) in the previous chapter, and I want to give it some well-deserved space now. EFT is one of the most accessible and effective ways I've learned to activate the parasympathetic nervous system. Not only can it calm us, it gives us the power to overcome negative thought spirals and integrate experiences that unsettle us, diminish our power, or otherwise hold us back.

Some people learn to practice EFT with the guidance of a teacher, but you can absolutely learn to do it yourself if you can move your arms. If not, a trusted caregiver could learn to tap for you, following your instructions.

Based on Chinese medicinal principles, EFT involves tapping your fingers on points in the body. These points correspond with the body's jing-luo or energy meridians (I like to think of them as our energy highway system) in the head, face, torso, and hands—some of the same points used in acupuncture.

Tapping can be done silently but is often paired with a script designed to help you let go of resistance to a feeling or message that may be causing you pain or anxiety, then move beyond it with affirmations that invite feelings of security, calmness, confidence, or empowerment.

When you first practice EFT, you'll feel silly. Everybody does. But the results soon quash the self-consciousness. Tapping is one of the only things that helps me return to sleep after a heart-pounding 3:00 am wakeup. (Many thanks to Amelia Jones, the teacher who introduced me to EFT!)

If you want to give it a try, here are the EFT points I was taught to use and a sample script to use when you're experiencing a spike of anxiety. I usually say each affirmation at least two times, but you can let your intuition guide you on how long you choose to tap each meridian.

1. Crown of the head: *"Even though I feel anxious right now, I completely love and accept myself."* You may wish to say this for all the meridians on your first tapping cycle to "clear the cache" and help yourself transition to a calmer state.

2. Inside of the eyebrows (two hands, either side of the bridge of your nose): *"Anxiety is temporary, and I won't always feel this way."*

3. Outside of the eyebrows (two hands, next to your temples): *"I am not my anxiety."*

4. Under the eye (two hands, like you're patting your eye bags): *"I am entitled to safety and happiness."*

5. Upper lip (one hand, under your nose): *"My body knows how to feel calm and centered."*

6. Chin crease (one hand, under your lower lip): *"I can help myself calm down wherever I need to."*

7. Chest (two hands, under your collarbones): *"I release all unnecessary tension from my body."*

8. Solar plexus (one or two hands, where your rib cage comes together): *"My heart is a reservoir of peace."*

9. Underarms (one or two hands, reach across your body, and tap where your bra strap would be if you were wearing a bra): *"I am ready to relax."*

10. Wrists (tap your wrists together): *"I am safe to let anxiety go."*

11. Back of the hand (below where the ring and pinky fingers meet): *"I am safe to invite serenity in."*

12. Side of the hand (below your pinky joint): *"I am safe."*

Repeat through two or three cycles or as many as you feel you need.

 To hear an audio version of this tapping script, visit **bigsober-energy.com/reader-bonuses.**

Singing and Laughing

You've read previously about the amplified power of affirmations due to the resonant power of our voices. Saying something out loud sends vibrations out into the universe that previously did not exist. Anyone who ever bottled up a feeling and then finally got it off their chest knows that speaking can radically change your physiology.

The same is true of singing and laughing; they create vibrations. We associate these activities with expression and joy, which means we can use singing and laughing to help reset our brains in the wake of having the emotional wind knocked out of us.

Belting out a song you connect with feels good. The shower, the car, the kitchen—doesn't matter. Just sing. Commit to your performance, and give yourself permission to laugh at yourself for being extra.

Laughter is another magical reset button. I keep an "LOL" folder of memes and videos on my phone to look at when I feel myself holding on to something that upsets me. If I can watch cats pushing water glasses off tables, I can usually start to let some shit go.

Dancing

Winner of "Most Fun Integration Technique" is...dancing!

In addition to my meme folder, I have a special playlist on my phone called "Songs to Get Out of Your Head." There are no ballads or meditation tracks on this playlist. It is completely devoid of depth. It is a "bops only" zone.

STGOOYH doesn't get played very often. It's kind of a "break glass in case of emergency" type of thing. It comes out when I'm feeling low and need to shake up my energy quickly.

Despite my love of slow, deliberate, micro-movements, sometimes you need to jump around and shake your ass. Like *really* shake it.

There are other playlists. Some make cleaning the house go faster. Some encourage me to walk my dog a little longer. I have one for moving with my eyes closed based entirely on how I feel inside (a true "dance like no one's watching" experience, and I *hope to god* no one is).

Joyful, intuitive movement can be a lifesaver, either as a way to spice up mundane tasks, stimulate a quick head change when you're in a funk, or otherwise bring yourself back to baseline. Dancing releases pleasure hormones, and hormones are basically drugs. So if you're processing something that makes you feel blue, fuck drinking. Try Dua Lipa instead.

CHAPTER 8

TRUTH BE TOLD

"Lies only strengthen our defects. They don't teach any-
thing, help anything, fix anything, or cure anything."

— JOSÉ N. HARRIS

One of the most painful things for me to admit about the height of my drinking days is how often I lied. On a daily basis, I told dozens of lies without even thinking about it. Here are some of the greatest hits:

- "I only had three drinks!" when I drank seven.
- "I don't feel that bad," when I was so hungover, I wanted to die.
- "So-and-so is waaaay worse than me," when I knew full well I was the drunkest person at the party.

These were lies of deflection and denial, the kind told by someone who is trying desperately to control the narrative. If I were honest about how much I was drinking, how terrible I felt most of the time, and how much of a hot mess I was, I would have had to do something about it. And I just wasn't ready.

In most cases, I'm willing to bet that everyone involved in these conversations knew I was full of shit. It was pretty rare that anyone pressed me when I glossed over my behavior or fabricated a version of reality in which I wasn't spiraling out of control.

I get it. I've done the same thing for people I could tell were hurting. Sometimes, I still do, and it makes me wonder: When we pretend to believe someone's lies, is that lying, too?

The "nothing to see here" lies were far from the worst of it. I was sneaky and dishonest in other ways. Swearing I was home when I was out partying. Saying I hadn't driven drunk when I had. Pretending I had food poisoning when, in reality, I was too ravaged from the night before to go to work (a lie I sometimes stretched for two or more days to make it more "believable").

Maintaining the facade of a functional life when you have substance use disorder is similar to putting on a tacky magic show. Behind the scenes, there's an intricate apparatus rigged to create the illusion; onstage, the smokescreen must remain thick enough that no one can see you frantically stacking decks and pulling levers.

Despite the enormous amount of orchestration, most people don't believe the magic in those shows is real. And, after a while, most of them don't believe our lies, either.

Much ink has been spilled on the topic of lying and honesty and integrity. Do we degrade ourselves a little each time we lie—even if we never get caught? Are lies told out of self-preservation or kindness as bad as lies told to manipulate or harm?

I am not a moral philosopher, but I was raised with a strong sense of integrity (even if it didn't always translate into my actions). Every time I found myself debating the question about how "bad" it was to tell a given lie, I knew my internal compass was busted: I had strayed far away from the truth of who I thought I was—who I used to be.

By telling myself I wasn't hurting anyone with my lies, I forgot that *I* am someone. Moreover, I was hurting myself *to maintain the facade necessary to keep hurting myself.*

The only way to change this dynamic was to begin seeing myself as valuable enough to want to protect. The only way to see myself that way was to actually respect the person I saw in the mirror.

And the only way to do *that* was to stop lying.

INTENTION

Finding your way back to yourself is easier in song lyrics than in reality, but recalibrating your internal compass *is* possible. One way to speed up the process is to set your intention and commit to telling the truth. All the time.

When I was getting certified to teach meditation, my own teacher Dina Kaplan shared with our class an article she had written called "Two Years No Lies."[21] In it, she described unintentionally taking a vow of honesty at a meditation retreat and being shocked by how challenging it was to stick to.

"I was shocked at how often I lied to people about little things, unimportant items that I easily could have been truthful about," she recalls in the article. "It's almost like I had a reflex to lie only about things I had no reason to lie about. Stamping this out was primarily logistical, like learning a new language."

Saying only things that are true sounds easier than it is. Even if you think you're an honest person, once you make this commitment, you will notice how easily white lies slip out of your mouth. It's almost as if our brains are programmed to avoid bumpy or unpleasant truths and find the smoothest path—even if it's paved with lies.

If substance use disorder has trained your brain to seek pleasure and veer away from pain, your preference for the smoother path is likely already the default. This can make the transition to truth-telling feel even rockier, but it also offers you a shortcut to trusting yourself more, something many of us in recovery struggle with.

One of the things I always remembered about Dina's article was that after giving up lying, she noticed that she liked herself more.

"In many ways [telling the truth] is an act of self-love, and it becomes a moral barometer that affects other actions, too," she explains. "Subconsciously, it holds you to your values."

MEDITATION

One of my favorite ways to use affirmations is to remind myself why the hell I'm doing something. They keep me motivated and accelerate my results because my subconscious is primed to look for evidence that what I'm doing works.

In addition to a regular mindful meditation practice, affirmations can be an excellent way to support your commitment to truth-telling. Some of my favorites include:

> *It is safe for me to be honest with myself and others.*
>
> *The more honest I am, the more peace I invite into my life.*
>
> *I release the impulse to lie and forgive myself for lying in the past.*
>
> *I embrace the truth and trust that it will serve my highest good.*

Another way your meditation practice can support greater honesty is to visualize the lies leaving your life and creating space for more joy, connection, and peace. Have fun with it. Imagine the lies have a weaselly personality and a grubby little face. Perhaps they look like Mitch McConnell. (Mine absolutely look like Mitch McConnell.)

Pick a departure for your lies that feels satisfying to you. Slingshot them out into the atmosphere or simply show them the door. Then, imagine a flood of well-being washing over you, filling in the places corroded by deception with a warm, golden light. If you catch yourself in a lie, you can use this visualization in the moment to reset your energy.

ALIGNED ACTION

At a basic level, the aligned action step for this one could boil down to simply: *Don't lie, ever.* But it's a little more complicated than that.

For example, in early sobriety, there may be good reasons to lie. Say you're trying to string a few alcohol-free days together, but the people you see on those days either aren't supportive or aren't the people you feel like talking to about your decision. Most recovery mentors and coaches will tell you it's perfectly fine to say, "I have to drive," "I'm on medication," "I don't feel well," or "My dentist could only see me at 11:00 pm tonight." Say whatever it takes to avoid a conversation that could derail you.

Most recovery mentors and coaches will also tell you it is not sustainable to keep your sobriety to yourself long-term. Being secretly sober after being famously boozy is not realistic. Even if it was, it would require hiding a big part of yourself—like *forever*—and we're trying to get free of that exhausting bullshit, right? Right.

However, during those first tender weeks when you feel like Bambi trying to figure out how to walk, I am firmly on team "Do Whatever You Need to Do." That includes fibbing to get people off your back.

Pick your parameters

Even outside of early sobriety, there are different kinds of lies and reasons to lie. Are you lying to protect someone's safety or to make yourself look better? Are you lying to keep a surprise party secret or because you don't want to get in trouble for something you did wrong?

If your sister is being held hostage and her kidnappers ask if you came alone to drop the ransom money, should you tell them you brought the cops? Probably not.

If your best friend has a baby and gives it a horrible name that you would never, in a million billion years, curse a child with, are you going to volunteer your hatred for her choice? I wouldn't, but you do you.

So, yeah. Pick your parameters. But don't get caught up in the mental gymnastics of finding loopholes that make lying "okay." That defeats the purpose. Default to the truth. Even if people's feelings are at stake, you can find kind, constructive ways of telling people what you think or why you made a certain decision.

You don't have to commit to radical honesty, but a minimum commitment of only speaking words that are true is a good place to start.

Notice your patterns

Once you practice this aligned action, you'll notice the corners of your life where lies tend to cluster like dust bunnies.

Dina, for example, caught herself having the impulse to lie about why she was late. Instead, she would say, "I'm sorry I'm late, but I didn't manage my time properly, and I left late to meet you. I apologize, and I'll try not to do it again."

People were often taken aback by her simple, direct honesty, but they respected it.

After our patterns reveal themselves, coming up with honest explanations for things we used to frequently lie about is the next level. Over time, you'll have to either become skilled at delivering the explanation or change your behavior to avoid the situation in the first place.

Removing the convenience of lying forces you to take the higher road, and I would argue that the high road gets you where you want to go faster.

Turn the honesty inward

After you've practiced your commitment of telling the truth to others, I'm willing to bet you'll start noticing how often you lie to yourself. Thanks to our old friend neuroplasticity, your brain will hiccup when you minimize, gloss over, or otherwise deceive yourself in an effort to avoid doing or facing something you know you need to.

This is a good thing, but it can feel like a bad thing in the moment. Our brains are good at protecting us. In many cases, that protection is a trauma response. Facing false narratives can be scary, but it's necessary for us to truly liberate ourselves. Being honest about things we did when we were drinking can stir up a lot of shame, but that shame was already there. Shining a light on it is the best opportunity we have to let it dry up and float away.

If self-trust is a particularly acute issue in your recovery, consider adding a weekly journaling practice focused on honesty. Respond to the following questions:

What was the most difficult moment of honesty for me this week?

When did I change my behavior to avoid lying?

How would I describe my current level of integrity?

The purpose of this exercise is not to judge or rate yourself but simply to reflect and learn from your experience.

INTEGRATION

Committing to tell the truth is already an integrative practice; as Dina says, it's like learning a new language. Honesty becomes part of your life on a minute-by-minute basis. This will fundamentally change your outlook and your energy.

If you notice an inner truth coming up for you that you're not ready to face, I highly recommend working with a therapist to navigate and integrate these experiences. Forcing yourself to handle them alone can interfere with the integration process or result in unnecessary self-punishment.

You deserve support as you adjust to walking the path of honesty.

ENERGY BOUNDARIES: NAVIGATING OTHER PEOPLE

I have read not one but two recovery books that include chapters titled "Hell Is Other People." I understand why. When we attempt to change our lives, it is almost inevitable that some people around us will resist that change or even try to sabotage it. They may not be malevolent people, but they have grown accustomed to a certain dynamic. They may resent that the dynamic has changed without their participation—even if it's clearly what's best for you.

It is also the case that we may not have been the greatest child, sibling, partner, employee, citizen, or friend while drinking or using. We may have some amends to make or learning to do when it comes to creating and maintaining healthy connections. But the good news is navigating friends and family sober is a skill you can practice. The practices in this section will help you do this. Greater intimacy and stronger relationships are waiting.

CHAPTER 9

WHAT MAKES ME HAPPY?

"Whatever is bringing you down, get rid of it."

— TINA TURNER

When I was a child, my parents read me the Mr. Men book series by Roger Hargreaves. If you've never read them, the premise is simple: Each "Mr." embodies a single characteristic that defines his life. Mr. Messy lives in squalor. Mr. Nosey is all up in everyone's business. Mr. Grumble complains about everything (until a wizard turns him into a pig—because that makes total sense and is definitely a cure for grumpiness).

And then there's Mr. Happy, who spends his day strolling around Happyland, smiling and cheering up Mr. Miserable.

Now, baby me was *obsessed* with these books—but not with Mr. Happy. I didn't get him. A story about a guy who walked around smiling all the time rang hollow to me. It felt suspicious. And what was the moral supposed to be, anyway? Just be...happy?

I preferred the Mr. Men whose one defining characteristic created tension in their lives. My favorite was Mr. Quiet, who lived in Loudland where he was constantly startled by noisy neighbors who never listened to him. His life was defined by what made him *un*happy. He spent most of his time hiding in his home, the only place he could find reprieve from the jarring, overwhelming world.

Looking back, it's funny to me how strongly I identified with Mr. Quiet and what a straight line can be drawn between my own Mr. Quiet tendencies and my drinking.

Did I feel invisible and unheard? Yes, until a couple of glasses of wine emboldened me to raise my voice.

Did the cacophony of the world make me harrowingly anxious? Yes, until the weighted blanket of alcohol draped itself over my brain.

Did I flee every scene that made me feel uncomfortable? Pretty much, and if I couldn't flee, I'd drink until I didn't care anymore.

My life was also defined by what made me unhappy, or rather, by avoiding it: seeking whatever would numb my feelings of anxiety and self-doubt. So, for years, I conflated happiness with whatever made me drunk or high.

Alcohol and drugs were how I knew to manipulate the serotonin levels in my brain. For a long time, I believed I was quite good at this manipulation, and I was. But as anyone with substance use disorder knows, that game only lasts for so long.

As time went on and it took more and more booze or pills or whatever to bring me back to baseline, happiness became an apparition—chemical or otherwise. Even as a kid, happiness had never felt that real to me. During my drinking years, it felt like a straight-up fairytale—a mythical place inhabited by two-dimensional people whose bodies were made out of yellow circles with hands where their ears should have been.

So it was quite a surprise to me when, as a newly sober person, a meditation teacher instructed me to "pay attention to the things that make you happy." His words sounded foreign. It alarmed me that I had no idea what made me happy. Moreover, I had no idea how to *find out* what made me happy.

I knew what made other people happy, but it was becoming clear to me that accommodating the emotional lives of everyone around me did not count as caring for my own.

I knew I loved my husband and would do anything for him because I wanted to, not because I was scared not to. Was that because he made me happy?

I ran this experiment over and over in my mind, replacing "husband" with the other precious things in my life I hadn't completely fucked up or alienated. Question marks remained.

Eventually, two things happened that helped solve the mystery of my missing happiness.

One, I remained sober long enough that my brain chemistry started to balance itself out. My cravings became less intense. My shame abated. I was meditating and sleeping better. I don't know if I was back to baseline because I didn't know what that was for me anymore. But being released from the hangover cycle gave me back some emotional stability—relief in and of itself.

The other thing that happened is that, as I began practicing mindfulness more organically, I became more attuned to how I felt throughout the day. I'd find myself automatically checking in with my emotions during periods of stress or chaos, and noticing when I needed a bit of distance to avoid sinking into a craving. As these self-check-ins became habitual, I was also able to catch sight of moments that made me feel especially joyful, peaceful, or at ease.

They were there! I *was* capable of happiness and I probably always had been. The key was learning to recognize it in day-to-day moments rather than chase after it via dramatic disruptions in brain chemistry.

INTENTION

Let's go back to why it's so critical to know what sparks your joy.

The reason I push so hard on registering happiness is not that I think happiness should be our ultimate goal. I promise, I'm not trying to sneak in a good-vibes-only message. *Let's hear it for embracing the full spectrum of human emotions!*

No, the reason is that being at ease in our lives and free to show up and be present as the most authentic version of ourselves is one of the most beautiful and important shifts we can make in sobriety. But to do this, we must exercise discretion. We must pursue the things that fill us up, inspire us, and align with our being—and that requires knowing what those things are.

The pursuit of this knowledge must be the focus of our intention; without it, we won't have the data we need to create the sober life we truly want.

You may feel uncomfortable focusing on yourself in this way. If you were raised as a woman, it almost certainly goes against your conditioning. But don't be afraid to be radically self-centered as you work to overcome the discomfort. You're not leaving anyone behind (and anyone who accuses you of such probably belongs in the rear-view mirror). Knowing yourself and your desires will make you a better community member, partner, and friend.

MEDITATION

Any and all meditation practices will aid you in the quest to better understand your emotional weather forecast. The very first practice I outlined in Chapter 5 drives home the "why," but it bears repeating: Once you get in the habit of observing your mind during meditation, you will naturally start to observe your feelings and reactions throughout the day. Noticing when you register happiness offers you the opportunity to choose people, activities, and circumstances that spark joy whenever possible.

A second meditation technique I find useful for this practice is visualizing myself in a setting or scenario that might be causing me anxiety and picturing it going exactly as I would want it to go. I decide how I want to show up, how I want others to treat me, and how I want to feel. When I find myself in the real-life scenario, I match my energy to my visualization.

It would be a lie (and you already know I try not to do that!) to say my experience always matches my mental pregame show. But even when it doesn't, I am prepared to ask myself, "Is this okay with me? Does this square with my boundaries?" Most of the time, the answer is yes. I can either change my experience or adjust my expectations without putting my needs on the back burner.

But if I'm not feeling it for any reason, I leave. Denying people access to you = the ultimate boundary.

Pro tip: Knowing you can leave and viewing it as a viable option is helpful when weighing the benefits of attending social events in early sobriety!

Many scenarios in sobriety will tax you, and that's okay. Meditation will help you parse out where the resistance is coming from. Is it an indicator of growth and worth pushing through? Or is your intuition telling you to sit this one out and rest?

ALIGNED ACTION

I've already explained my feelings on positivity for positivity's sake. And while relying solely on the "power of positive thinking" to change our lives is problematic (and ineffective), the idea is not completely without merit. I *do* believe that thoughts can change our feelings and feelings can change our behaviors, and behaviors can change our lives. So, with the caveats about privilege and oppression and needing to take action still withstanding, yes, changing your thoughts can change your life. But do those thoughts have to be *positive* to lead to improvements?

The aligned action step I'm about to teach you is a prime example of how defaulting to the word "no" can create positive energy shifts by removing obstacles and opening doors. The actions themselves may feel negative, but the results create space for significantly more freedom and ease. What could be more positive than that?

I've run across versions of this practice in different places over the years, and under several different names. Here, I'm going to call it the Life Edit. The Life Edit urges us to become brutally discerning curators of our calendars, our relationships, our experiences, and our obligations.

Here's how it works.

Step 1: Make a list of everything in your life that you feel you must do: your obligations.

Be expansive. Include carpools you drive, birthday dinners you've been invited to, bills you're expected to pay, work events you're asked to attend, etc.

If your list is long, you may want to group it by category, such as family, social, financial, employment, spiritual, and any others that apply to you. Your categories might look different depending on your lifestyle. If you're not sure what they are, brainstorm the list first, then look for themes or patterns to emerge.

Once you've completed your list, make two columns, one on either side. Label the one on the left, "Urgency," and the other, "Desire."

Urgency	Obligation	Desire

Step 2: Next, go through your list, category by category.

Evaluate each item for its true level of urgency. What is the worst thing that will happen if you don't do this thing?

Some things are truly urgent. You must pay your rent or mortgage, or you will not have a place to live. You must feed your children and pets if you have them. If you're newly sober, attending meetings, coaching, or therapy sessions is likely non-negotiable. But it's worth taking a second and third look at this list because things that might seem urgent at first glance become less so upon closer examination.

For example, you might have been invited to a friend's baby shower. This feels urgent at first because the expectant parent is your friend and the arrival of a baby is a joyful event in their life. But how urgent is it *really*? Are you throwing the shower at your house? Are you the lead planner? If the answer is no, then your presence is a nice-to-have for the shower recipient, not a necessity. No one will die or be harmed if you don't go. Feelings might be temporarily hurt, but will probably heal quickly if you send a nice gift or a card expressing sincere well-wishes and offering to deliver a meal. In reality, attending a baby shower is likely of low-to-no urgency.

What about a dental cleaning (if one is fortunate enough to have dental insurance)? Not super urgent, probably, because it is preventative and routine, but a good thing to do regularly for self-care and overall health. I would categorize this as medium urgency. It could be moved or skipped once without a major consequence but probably should not be stricken from the list altogether.

Urgency	Obligation	Desire
Medium	Dental Cleaning	
Low	Baby Shower	

Step 3: Ask yourself: How do I feel?

This is where you allow your energy and your intuition to lead the way. When you read each item on the list, what emotions arise? Think of this as the Marie Kondo-ing of your schedule. Does the event or obligation spark joy? Dread? Some emotion in between?

Let's look at our examples again. It is possible that, for some people, the idea of attending a baby shower would spark joy. I am not one of those people. I am not a parent, I have no infant-care advice to dispense, and the idea of spending hours watching someone unwrap Diaper Genies and bibs is akin to one of the more painful rings of hell. For me, that particular obligation is both low urgency and low desire.

Now, a dental cleaning might be torture for some people, but personally, I love the way my teeth feel when they are freshly scraped and polished. Plus, I enjoy the positive reinforcement I get for being a consistent flosser (*thanks, sobriety!*). So, in my twisted world, dental cleaning would be of medium urgency, high desire.

Urgency	Obligation	Desire
Medium	Dental Cleaning	High
Low	Baby Shower	Low

If you're more of a visual processor, you could even plot your obligations on a quadrant graph, like this.

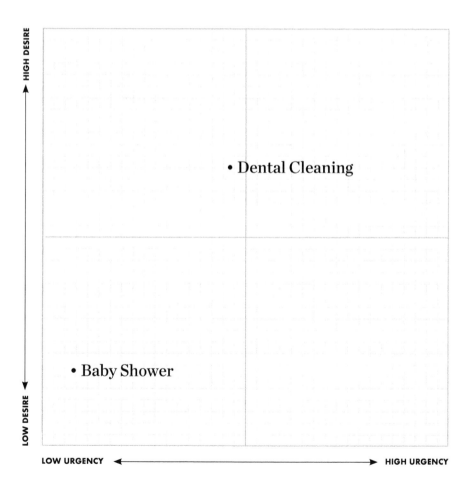

Step 4: Go through your list (or your chart) and cross out anything with low or medium urgency that isn't high desire.

This step is terrifying at first but, eventually, becomes the fun part.

This might feel extreme, but think of it as counter-conditioning. Those of us who were raised as women are especially susceptible to feeling like we must agree to anything that is asked of us (explicitly or implicitly), and that once we say *yes,* we must follow through, even if we don't want to. Some of these expectations are projected upon us by people currently in our lives, but many of them come from past relationships, cultural norms, or defaulting to what will cause the least amount of conflict (a totally legitimate choice when we are unsafe or exhausted).

The simplest way to explain this step is to say *no* to everything that isn't a *hell yes.* Setting aside obligations that cannot be postponed or skipped without jeopardizing health, safety, and security, the only items left on your list should be things that light you up.

Urgency	Obligation	Desire
Medium	Dental Cleaning	High
~~Low~~	~~Baby Shower~~	~~Low~~

Moreover, by removing the things that don't light you up, you create more space to add in things that do. For example, if you love to read or hike or you've always wanted to learn a language but felt you didn't have time for those things, you can create that time. Ask another parent to drive the carpool. Redirect some grocery money to a meal delivery service.

"Can I do that?" you might be asking yourself. The answer is, it depends on your circumstances. If you are a single parent working three jobs, there may be very little you can trim. But that makes the result even more powerful; removing even a few obligations from an overwhelming life can add a tremendous boost of energy, no matter how busy you are.

If cultivating your own happiness is a priority, I highly recommend this exercise, even if it's a bit uncomfortable. And it probably will be. Not everyone is going to be happy about it, namely people who are used to having unlimited access to your time, attention, and energy. But *their potential unhappiness is not more important than your happiness.*

INTEGRATION

Saying *no* to everything that's not an immediate *yes* is a hard habit to establish and, realistically, it can make for some awkward conversations.

My favorite tool for integrating this energy shift and making conversations a little smoother is to never agree to anything in the moment. Ever. Once you know that's your default, you can practice different ways of saying it, and you'll never again hear yourself agreeing to do something you'd rank below colonoscopy prep on the "desire" scale.

It looks like this. You run into your boss in the hallway. She says, "Oh, by the way, can you set up the going-away party for Sasha in the breakroom on Friday? I'm totally swamped."

Rather than say *yes* and stew about it all week, simply say, "I'll look at my schedule and get back to you." If you are too busy or you don't want to do it (and it's not in your job description, which would up the urgency), send your boss an email explaining that it's not a good week to take on extra tasks. You don't have to go into an exhaustive explanation; just say you can't do it.

Over time, these practices become easier and thus more integrated for two reasons.

One, the boundaries we build around our time and energy begin to set themselves. People will no longer ask you to do the things they don't want to do because they no longer perceive you as a bottomless receptacle for their unwanted tasks.

Two, as you become clearer about the life you want, it becomes easier to only say *yes* to the things that enrich that vision. You begin to value, and thus protect, your time and energy more fiercely and consistently. You create the energetic conditions that support a life that makes you want to say *yes!*

And, before we close out this chapter, if you were worried about the fate of poor Mr. Quiet, I want you to know that his life turns into a *yes!* life in the end. And, ironically, the hero in Mr. Quiet's story turns out to be (*drumroll please*) Mr. Happy!

Mr. Happy sends Mr. Quiet a letter and invites him to visit Happyland. Once he arrives, Mr. Quiet gets a job at the library, where everyone has to be quiet all the time. And guess what? He's so fucking happy. He says yes to quietness *and* to happiness. He changes the conditions of his life. And even though he is a little gold circle with arms sticking out where his ears should be, I always feel so overjoyed for this fictional oddball at the end of that book. In a world where loudness always seems to win, there's a place for Mr. Quiet and for me. We may not be able to "choose happiness" like Mr. Happy, but we can learn to look for it and put ourselves in its path.

CHAPTER 10

HOW TO PLUG AN ENERGY LEAK

"Where attention goes, energy flows."

— JAMES REDFIELD

It's a Tuesday. You know you have an appointment with your therapist later that day, but you can't remember when it is. You log into your email to check the handy confirmation message, but before you find it, you see another email from a newsletter you vaguely remember subscribing to. The subject line reads, "All your new favorites are waiting for you!"

My favorite new whats? You click on it. It takes you to a post listing the latest and greatest camping gear. It's riddled with affiliate links and videos. One of them is a review of a tent you've been eyeing. You click on it. Before the video even plays, you see an ad for the tent's manufacturer. You click on it and go to their website. Damn, they're expensive!

You wonder if the tent is available cheaper on eBay. You open a browser window, but the website seems to know you're leaving. It pops open a window promising you 20 percent off if you subscribe to *their* newsletter. You attempt to simultaneously subscribe to the camping newsletter while searching for the tent on eBay.

But before you can even scope out the minimum bid, you get a notification on your phone; someone sent you a DM on Instagram. You click on it. It's the tent! It found you! Isn't that wonderful? Or is it creepy? Never mind, now it's *25* percent off! You wonder if the eBay seller can match that. But before you go back to your browser, you decide to take a quick peek at Instagram. You see a Reel your friend posted in their stories. You click on it...

Two hours later, you realize you missed your therapy appointment.

I wish this were a fictional example, but I have some version of this experience on a regular basis. And I don't even have ADD. But you don't need an attention deficit diagnosis to find your attention completely hijacked in this day and age. There is a billion-dollar industry devoted to capturing your attention online and directing it toward products you are likely to buy.

The attention economy, as it's often called, works by masterfully stringing together breadcrumbs through inboxes, browsers, websites, and media platforms that are ostensibly "free." I put free in quotes because, of course, they are not free. You are paying for them with your eyes, your time, your attention, and with the purchases you ultimately make because you followed the breadcrumbs that were set out specifically for you. Capitalism feeds on attention. You are the product.

I bring this up for two reasons.

One, the mechanisms of the attention economy offer a perfect metaphor for how energy work functions. Let's take the camping company as an example. The company's intention is for you to buy the latest model of their super expensive tent. To make that happen, they create the conditions necessary to capture your attention—and your energy— and move it toward that goal. They do this by making sure their ads appear everywhere you spend time online and then reaching out to you directly once they know they've caught your eye. And they repeat this behavior until you either block their ads or buy the damn thing.

Whether you consider it insidious or genius or both, this kind of sticky marketing makes a strong case for the power of repetition. We can use this power to protect ourselves and our energy from the manipulative, capitalism-driven attention economy. This is easier said than done; if we are not extremely deliberate about what we pay attention to, it's easy to inadvertently begin leaking energy in directions that do not align with our vision and values.

You can also build your own attention economy. This brings us to reason two.

As our friend James Redfield tells us, where attention goes, energy flows. How do we capture our own attention? By deliberately creating reminders and invitations to point our laser in a direction that enhances our energy and our power, rather than dilutes or diminishes it.

We'll talk more about how to do this on a practical, day-to-day basis—including steps that can help corral your attention online—in Chapters 11 and 12. But your online attention is not your only hot commodity; your interpersonal attention and energy are, too.

Protecting your interpersonal energy is the foundation for growing the skills to protect yourself and your energy in any setting, so we'll start here.

INTENTION

Your intention when it comes to energy protection might be different from mine and from anyone else's. The things that drain and threaten your energy are unique to your life. But there are a few universals that can help ground any protection practice.

If you're reading this book sequentially (and it's okay if you're not!), you've already learned about the value of asking yourself how you feel, listening to your body, and paying attention to the things that make you happy. Energy protection takes these practices to the next level, so at the very least consider setting an intention to grow your power and skills in service of yourself and your recovery.

If you're an empath or a highly sensitive person, another intention that may benefit you is learning to differentiate between your energy versus energy that is "hitching a ride" or being projected onto you.

This is huge, in part because people raised as women are conditioned to pay attention to other people's energy, in many cases out of self-preservation.

Moreover, newly sober people are regularly asked to absorb other people's anxieties about their own drinking and fears of being judged for not abstaining. That is a *lot* to carry on top of navigating your own anxieties and insecurities without the dulling effect of alcohol. Focusing your intention on distinguishing between what is yours to carry and what is other people's shit to work through is an extremely helpful starting place.

Finally, another universally helpful intention is to get good at identifying energy vampires. If you're not familiar with that term, an energy vampire is exactly what it sounds like: a person who sucks energy and needs constant attention to function.

We may love the energy vampires in our lives. We can have compassion for them. We may have even been one of them when we were drinking or using. But the fact is, if we consistently leave someone's company feeling depleted, then we won't have energy for ourselves or for the other people in our lives.

As uncomfortable as it is to recognize, it's usually not a coincidence that energy vampires attach themselves to people who don't have great protection in place. They are attracted to shaky boundaries, even if they're not consciously trying to violate them.

Alcohol, of course, weakens our boundaries. This means vampirism may ramp up when we get sober, and our boundaries become firmer. People we used to gleefully and recklessly exchange energy with can become increasingly needy once we begin rationing the supply. (Conversely, they may pull their energy away, and we may find ourselves growing our own sets of fangs!)

A worldview oriented toward generosity and seeing the best in people is not mutually exclusive with recognizing and avoiding energy vampirism. This intention simply boils down to: Know what you have to give, and don't give a drop more.

Many people who practice vipassana or insight meditation talk about coming into a deep sense of *knowing* the longer they practice. As you distance your consciousness from the hamster wheel of your mind, that knowing allows you to gauge more and more accurately how much energy you have to give and what reserves you may need to protect. All forms of meditation will help you activate this form of protection.

Another type of meditation I often rely on to enhance this knowing is a visualization to balance my energy centers or points where energy channels converge. In the Hindu and Tantric Buddhist traditions, these points are referred to as chakras.

My understanding of chakras is decidedly Western; because of this, I am more comfortable using the term energy center. I don't speak Sanskrit and cannot confidently claim to accurately represent the original spiritual intention of using chakras in energy work. With these caveats, I respectfully include here my simplified interpretation of a modern practice that is loosely based on what I have been taught about an ancient tradition.

Each energy center in the body connects with a different aspect of our lives and experiences; most modern Western spiritual teaching focuses on seven distinct energy centers and associates each with a color, although different Tantric traditions identify as many as 12, 16, 21, even up to 100 energy centers, both within and outside the body.[22]

Focusing on each energy center as you breathe allows you to tune in very specifically to what you feel and where you feel it (i.e., a sense of lethargy in your chest, a feeling of excitement in your stomach, or a sensation of heaviness in your legs). These sensations give us information about where we may need more or less stimulation, relaxation, or another type of attention to keep our energy balanced and flowing.

Many people directly ascribe physical ailments to unbalanced energy. For example, if you have something to say but don't feel comfortable expressing yourself, you may experience soreness or other symptoms in your throat.

This level of specificity is useful when you find your attention being drained or sucked in directions that don't serve your intention.

If you notice an energy disturbance, it could be that someone you've interacted with projected their bad attitude or misguided demands onto you. If you feel yourself leaking energy, it could be an imbalance caused by your misaligned focus pulling you in unhelpful directions.

Either way, the methodical, observational quality of this meditation can help.

As I said earlier, my cultural lineage does not include teaching about chakras. I encourage you to seek out different sources of information about energy centers and chakras written by teachers who are deeply familiar with Tantric, Vedic, and Buddhist traditions. I have included some of these resources at the end of the book.

Energy Center Visualization

Begin by sitting or lying down with your spine straight. Take three full breaths, then breathe normally. Focus on your inhales and exhales.

Next, bring your attention to the base of your spine, your root energy center, and the source of groundedness and security. Visualize a red spiral gently spinning inside your pelvis. Notice if the spiral moves easily and naturally or if that area of your body feels blocked in any way. Breathe, and allow yourself to be surrounded by a red aura. Use your breath to invite the root energy through your body.

Repeat this process for the remaining six energy centers:

1. The sacral energy center is just below your navel. It is the source of your creativity and is commonly associated with the color orange.

2. The solar plexus energy center is located where the two cages of your ribs meet in the middle of your torso. Usually depicted as yellow, it represents your divine essence and wholeness of being.

3. The heart energy center is higher up in your chest, and its aura is green. This is the center that rules connection and emotion.

4. The throat energy center is located exactly where you'd expect. Its color is light blue, and it is connected to communication and expression.

5. Between your brows is the third eye, a dark blue energy center associated with intuition and visualization.

6. Finally, the top of your head, or crown, is the center that connects you to universal energy or consciousness. In some traditions, it is white; in others, it is purple.

7. Depending on how much time I have to do this visualization, I will sometimes go through the energy centers several times, from bottom to top and top to bottom. Some people like to begin the day by waking up their energy centers from root to crown, and then "close them down" at night in the opposite order.

However you choose to practice this meditation, take your time. Tuning into your body can be very intense; not everyone will enjoy this or feel safe doing it. Once you feel the centers, you can't unfeel them. But if you're comfortable practicing it, this visualization can be an incredible source of information for you as well as a tool for finding greater protection, balance, and ease.

 To listen to a guided version of this visualization, visit **bigsoberenergy.com/reader-bonuses.**

ALIGNED ACTION

Protection is a huge subcategory of energy work, and one of the most frequently practiced. Ever seen someone throw salt over their shoulder? Protection. Horseshoe over the door? Protection. Knocking on wood? Protection. The list goes on, and with all the herbs and crystals and minerals and rituals and spells devoted to warding off harm, the possibilities you can choose are literally—and fantastically—endless.

The energy protection I teach leans heavily on visualization because it doesn't require special spaces, tools, or a lot of time. But if that modality doesn't come easily to you, don't despair. All of these suggestions can be done in verbal or sensory modes as well. It's also very likely that, as you get used to activating your energy in this way, you'll start to develop your own protection practices.

Rolling Up the Window

Take the practice I like to call "Rolling Up the Window." This is one I use when I find myself in a conversation with someone who attempts to cross my boundaries or moves the conversation in a direction I do not wish to go.

Because I am in the habit of asking myself how I feel and committed to protecting my energy, I act quickly when my brain registers the message "I want this to be over." I do this by visualizing a barrier rising up between the other person and me, as if I've pressed a button that closes a screen or a window between us.

I don't know what happens to my face or my body language when I do this because I can't see myself. I don't know if my appearance changes at all, but I know my energy changes because I can feel it. In almost all cases, the other person can feel it, too.

Even if the other person doesn't sense the shift, rolling up the window gives me the moment of separation I need to disengage. This might come in the form of a quick, "Excuse me, it's been lovely talking to you, but I need to attend to something." It might take the form of silently walking away. In most cases, it's something in between. But in any event, I rescue myself.

If visualizing the window is hard, you can simply say to yourself, "Rolling up the window. This is done," and feel a barrier materialize between you and the unwanted conversationalist.

Body Scan and Cord Cutting

A series of protection visualizations I love to recommend came from my training with Dr. Kate Tomas. I try to do them every night before falling asleep, although they can be activated at any time.

After you get into bed at night but before you doze off, take a moment to scan your body. This scan is similar to the energy center meditation but more rapid and less focused (although I love that meditation before bed if you have the mental space). Think of it as a ring of observation sliding down your body, like an invisible MRI machine without the banging and claustrophobia.

As you scan, notice where you're holding tension or any other evidence of poor circulation, stuck emotions, or energy buildup. Wherever you find it, pause for a moment and ask yourself: *Is this my energy or energy that has been projected onto me?*

Once you determine whether you have any hitchhiker energy weighing you down, attempt to locate the origin. Sometimes you won't be able to. In those cases, simply gather the energy into the center of your chest on an inhale, and send it back out to wherever it came from with your exhale.

But if you *do* know where the energy came from, you can engage in a mental cord-cutting exercise.

Say you had a bad interaction with a friend who accused you of lording your sobriety over them. You've checked in with yourself to make sure you don't, in fact, hold any feelings of superiority over this friend, but you found nothing. This is all them.

Now, imagine a cord running between you and your friend; the cord is the conduit. Deliberately and with love, send the energy back to your friend. Then, cut the cord. Finally, imagine winding the cord up, so it's tidy and safe and does not attract any new energy while you sleep.

Mirror Suit

The final visualization happens once you've sent all the hitchhiker energy back and tucked all the cords away. Now, imagine a mirrored catsuit covering your whole body. (If you don't like the catsuit, a mirrored blanket or a bubble works well, too.) The suit keeps your calm, relaxed energy safe and sound, while the mirrors reflect any external energy that may be swirling around while you sleep.

If the visualization doesn't come naturally, you can achieve the same effect by saying the words, "I return all unwanted energy to where it came from. I am entirely safe. I am entirely loved. I am entirely protected."

INTEGRATION

Like all energy work, protection is integrated through reflection and meaning-making. Maybe you found yourself in a situation where your energy was leaking but you felt powerless to stop it. Maybe there's a certain person you used to enjoy being around, but now you find them exhausting. Maybe you were more tempted than usual to drink. Maybe you even had a slip-up.

Whatever happened, give yourself grace and space to move through the experience without judgment. Recall the circumstances and any x-factors or variables that may have influenced why you felt the way you did. Glean what you can, and make a note of how you might approach the situation differently or avoid it altogether in the future. Then, let it go. You've taken the best the situation has to offer, which is learning. There's no need to dwell on the worst.

Integrating energy protection helps us learn to activate boundaries more quickly and decisively, especially in social situations where people are drinking. It becomes habitual over time. Eventually, we're so confidently protected, we exude Big Sober Energy wherever we go.

CHAPTER 11

HAPPY PLACE OR HELLSCAPE?

"Technology doesn't just do things for us. It does things to us, changing not just what we do but who we are."

— SHERRY TURKLE

Full disclosure: I have three Instagram accounts. That sounds like too many, I know. But hear me out.

I don't have three accounts because it benefits my social media "strategy." I have three accounts because it actually helps me use social media *less* than I would otherwise.

In the last chapter, we talked about the attention economy. Nowhere is that insidious beast better trained to suck your time and brain cells than on social media platforms. It is both the ultimate energy vampire and capitalism's current favorite tool. The scrolling, the liking, the algorithm that only shows you posts with the most drama-filled comments sections—all of these features are carefully designed to do three things:

1. Keep you on the platform (so you'll see more ads and buy more stuff)

2. Provoke your emotions (so you'll comfort yourself by buying more stuff) and

3. Keep you coming back over and over again (because scrolling and liking scratches an itch and, thus, exposes you to more ads.... you get the idea).

There is plenty of mud to sling when it comes to the ways that social media—and Facebook in particular—has allowed the proliferation of disinformation and hate. I'm not going to try to make the argument that the benefits of social media outweigh the devastating consequences for inclusive democracy. Social media is how huge swaths of the country came to believe COVID-19 was a hoax. But it has also brought #BlackLivesMatter and #MeToo into our consciousness and provided life-saving information and friendship to queer kids in rural areas. I can't throw it out altogether.

Regardless of how I or anyone feels about it, social media isn't going anywhere. Directly or indirectly, it's part of our lives. And because many of us give it our precious time and attention, it's also an energy tool that can either help or hinder us.

So, why three accounts? Doesn't that seem like an invitation to waste three times *more* energy?

The accounts break down like this: personal, podcast, recovery mentorship / book. Each account has a different purpose and follows a different set of accounts.

1. My personal account is strictly for looking at pictures of my friends' babies and pets.

2. The podcast account is where I used to post about new episodes when *Feminist Hotdog* was in production. Now, it's a tool to follow and share a lot of the political and cultural voices I came into contact with while making that show.

3. The recovery mentorship account is to share updates about my business, my new podcast, and expand on ideas related to the concept of Big Sober Energy!

Because each account has a narrow purpose, I keep the number of people I follow relatively small. This cuts waaaaay down on the scrolling because my feeds are set to suppress suggested content. (Yes, you can choose that option!)

On two out of three accounts, my usage is sporadic and mostly one-way: I post when I feel like it, scroll for a bit, share a few things that I think followers would like, and I'm out. I'm not super concerned about engagement. I am not Kylie Jenner, nor do I aspire to be.

If those Insta-boundaries seem aspirational, believe me, it took time (and a lot of muting, unfollowing, and letting go of expectations) to get here. Instagram is a hard place to be a small fish because you only get served content from accounts that have tons of followers and engagement. If that's not you, it can feel like you've lost yet another of life's popularity contests, when the truth is 91 percent of Instagram users have fewer than 10,000 followers.[23]

But if you can wrestle your self-worth away from the algorithm, there is a lot of power and inspiration to be gleaned from sober groups and accounts on social media. While there are toxic players in any arena, I have found sober Facebook and Instagram to be extremely welcoming places that enhance my recovery.

So, with that in mind, I want to share some suggestions for how to make social media work for you, with the giant caveat that you are a grown-ass person who gets to decide if you even want to make it work at all. If deleting TikTok off your phone is part of your path to liberation, I support you 100 percent. If scrolling keeps you from drinking, for fuck's sake, scroll away, baby!

INTENTION

The question I never asked myself (but should have) when I signed up for my first social media account (MySpace) was, "Why am I here?" If I had bothered to interrogate my motives, I would have discovered that I was there because everyone else was there and I didn't want to miss out. I wanted attention, the coolest wallpaper, and the hottest song. (MySpace let you choose the decor and soundtrack for your "space," which I very much miss.)

Those might not have been the noblest reasons to jump on a bandwagon, but they were my reasons, and they were fine. At the surface level, most of us are on social media because we want to know things about other people and we want them to know things about us. Some of us also want deeper connections. Some of us want to share things we create. Some of us want to show off how smart we are. Some of us, unfortunately, seem to want to hurt each other.

All of these reasons meet a need.

As you hone in on your intention for how (or if) you want to engage with social media, thinking about the need you are seeking to fulfill is an illuminating conversation to have with yourself. It opens the door to more questions like, "Is Instagram the best way for me to meet this need? Would I post this often if I felt like I was getting enough attention from my partner? Would I spend so much time scrolling if I felt more connected to my friends?"

Your reasons might not be my reasons, and that's okay. Celebrity distraction, fashion inspo, news analysis, and unlikely animal friendships are all valid reasons to log in! My nudge for you is simply to be as intentional as possible about how you spend your energy and what you invite into your consciousness. Simply asking, "Why am I here?" whenever you find yourself scrolling can be a huge energy shift in and of itself.

MEDITATION

If managing your time on social media is a goal for you, any mindfulness practice will help you curb your craving for content. This is true for two reasons.

One, social media is designed to suck us in and make us lose track of time; it is the opposite of mindfulness. Once you establish a regular meditation practice and start becoming more present in your daily life, you'll be less susceptible to getting swept away by an endless stream of 15-second videos.

Two, scrolling is part of a reward cycle, like drinking. You feel bored or anxious, so you pick up your phone, and suddenly your brain is lulled into a state of pleasant detachment. Once you recognize that, you can (if you want to!) use many of the same techniques to reroute the cycle that you use to ride out an impulse for alcohol or other drugs.

Here are a few meditation and mindfulness techniques you can access quickly in these moments.

- **Micro-meditation.** Take a few breaths to get centered and reconnect with your intention.

- **Rub the cartilage in your ears.** This helps your body relax by stimulating the vagus nerve.

- **Breathe into your belly.** Visualize breathing like a sleeping baby, and put your hand on your abdomen as it rises and falls.

- **RAIN.** An acronym for Recognize your feelings, Accept or Allow the experience, Investigate the circumstances, and Nurture or Non-identification with the emotions (i.e., you are not your thoughts or your feelings). You can read my full breakdown of RAIN in Chapter 5.

Social media cravings are unlikely to be as overwhelming as other cravings we experience in recovery, but that doesn't mean we should dismiss them. They are real and can be quite powerful. If you find you're having significant difficulty controlling your impulses around social media but can't quite give it up, you may want to add affirmations to your practice. Here are a few suggestions (although it is always more effective to write your own!).

I release the impulse to check Instagram (or Tik Tok or Facebook) every day.

I live my life in the present moment, not on the grid.

I am an excellent steward of my time, energy, and attention.

ALIGNED ACTION

Even if curbing your social media usage isn't a priority for you, you've probably heard most of the traditional advice. I'll summarize some of the highlights here in case you need a refresher. (I often do!)

- Use a time-limiting app like Anti Social or an internal timer (usually found in "settings") to alert you when you've reached your predetermined limit. If you don't want to get that technical, set a regular old timer. Anything that interrupts your use pattern can work, but the apps are more aggressive (and likely more effective for hard-core scrollers).

- Be consistent about rejecting and clearing cookies, using ad blockers, and browsing Incognito. This makes it harder for advertisers to track your interests and serve up gadgets and services that are likely to distract you.

- Get your phone out of your bedroom. Using any kind of screen late at night can negatively affect your sleep quality, and stuffing your psyche full of hot takes, breaking news, and filtered photos is the last thing you want to do to yourself first thing in the morning. Invest in an old-school alarm clock—but make sure it doesn't tick tick tick all night!

These suggestions are great, but they don't necessarily guide you in using social media in a way that might help you. So, I want to add a couple of aligned action steps that can connect how you want to show up in the world generally with how you want to show up online as you navigate your recovery.

Set a Scrolling Date

The first action is to schedule your social media time. I got this suggestion from writer Courtney Maum at a book talk she gave about her excellent memoir *The Year of the Horses*. It turns out even acclaimed writers get caught up in the social media fun-house mirror. It became clear to Courtney that her screen time felt less and less like a break and more like a series of self-inflicted blows to her ego. She and Instagram weren't working.

Instead of giving it up altogether, though, Courtney decided to schedule 30 minutes of social media time three days a week. This allowed her to keep up with author friends, family, thinkers she admired, and accounts she followed for fun. But she no longer spent hours comparing her appearance or her lifestyle to what she saw online. She simply didn't have time.

I love this approach to social media usage for two reasons. One, when you only allow yourself limited access to the feed, it forces you to be discerning about what you take time to post, read, and look at. A little built-in scarcity goes a long way toward streamlining your viewing.

I'm not usually a big proponent of self-limitation (alcohol and negative self-talk excepted, obviously). But in this case, the accompanying energy shift feels profound and worth it, especially since the algorithm will eventually respond and start showing you the stuff you've gone out of your way to see. It edits your feed for you—but in a good way. Instead of limitation, you end up with curation.

Embrace "Latergram"

The second action is to resist posting about your parties, vacations, shopping trips, brunches, etc. until *after* they've concluded.

Not everyone is a real-time poster, and if that's a habit you've broken or never developed, I applaud you. In the past, I could be having a magical experience in some exotic location and still feel compelled to duck into the Insta underworld and report my every move. For some reason, it felt important that my "followers" (groan) would know what I was seeing, hearing, or doing at that *exact* moment. Then, I'd pop back into my environment and try to reacclimate from looking at a 1080 px by 1080 px square to interacting with 3D life happening all around me. It was disorienting, isolating, and weird.

Having walked the path of a real-time poster and a reformed real-time poster, I can say with certainty that the latter is more relaxing. When you permit yourself to "be here now," the experience feels more authentic. You'll never get those moments back, so why not live them now and post about them later? Or not at all?

Waiting a day (or a week) or two to post also gives you time to sit with your experience and decide what you want to share and what should remain a memory for you and your loved ones.

I don't know about you, but I used to overshare a *lot* when I was intoxicated. Baring my soul or telling my dirty secrets to people I hardly knew felt like a way to establish the intimacy I craved. But in reality, it made me feel foolish and exposed. Being mindful about what and when we post is a way to reclaim some of the privacy and dignity we used to give away.

This is where the benefit comes in. You get to relive your brunch, your trip, or your walk in the woods. You get to decide what was special and joyful about it, whether you want to share it, and whether or not it might bring other people joy. That's a lovely conversation to get to have with yourself!

This last reason isn't nearly as fun to think about, but it's worth pointing out that waiting to post is safer. Do you really need every "friend" you've ever accepted knowing you're out of state for the weekend?

Don't Read the Comments, Don't Feed the Trolls

This one's pretty simple. Unless you are someone who derives tremendous joy and satisfaction from sparring online, don't fight on social media.

As someone with strong political beliefs, I have also walked both paths when it comes to this aligned action. It's tough because when people post misinformation or display their bigotry, I do feel compelled to comment, and sometimes I still do. But, in general, I try to save those conversations for face-to-face interactions when I can look into someone's eyes. The public nature of social media makes it too easy to center myself rather than the people who were most hurt by the comment.

These conversations are necessary, but I'm no longer convinced social media is the place to have them—at least not for me. And if you're in recovery and feeling at all fragile, I'm going to guess it isn't for you, either.

This doesn't apply only to racist classmates from high school. Recovery spaces, while generally welcoming, are not drama-free.

What I've learned is that not every online recovery space is for everyone. Like with any social network, it takes some time to find groups and accounts that match your recovery vibe.

For example, there are a *lot* of old-school, Christian recovery groups and accounts that simply do not speak to me, and that's fine. They are not for me, and I am certainly not for them. People in these groups post things I patently disagree with. They critique harm reduction tactics, believe it's necessary to reset your days if you have a slip-up, and insist that in order for anyone to get sober, they must accept the label of "addict" and surrender to a higher power.

That's a big "nope" from me on all counts.

But just because I don't agree with the folks in these groups doesn't mean I have to spend one millisecond trying to convince anyone that I'm right and they're wrong.

I don't have to do that because I've found incredible groups where I am fully supported and where I learn new things about myself and about recovery all the time.

And I have my own feed where I can talk as much or as little as I want about what I think is helpful and not helpful when it comes to staying sober. Hell, I wrote a whole-ass book about it!

Sometimes people come for me in the comments. I ignore them. I also use the "mute" and "unfollow" buttons liberally. If seeing someone in my feed doesn't bring me joy or at least make me think, they're gone. I'm not telling anyone what they can and can't post. There's no censorship happening. Facebook is not the library.

I may be choosing to live in a bubble, but I'm fine with that. Being careful about the energy I expose myself to is part of how I stay sober, and that's *way* more important than hurting someone's feelings because I unfollowed them. Social media is supposed to be beneficial and fun. As soon as it's not, you have the power to change whatever is not fun about it. Otherwise, what's the point?

INTEGRATION

Recovery at its essence is a process of returning to yourself, choosing yourself, and believing in yourself. You can use your new growth and skills to help manage a variety of compulsive behaviors, including reaching for your phone or getting lost in your feed, and that's rad. Finding a new relationship with social media that feels beneficial and friendly to your recovery is fantastic—whether it's a break, a breakup, or an ongoing romance.

But keep in mind that recovery is not static. Integrating your new social media relationship requires checking in with yourself and noticing how it makes you feel. Three months in, are you still choosing yourself? Has your online friend group changed, and did that change your feed? How do you feel when drinking memories pop up? Did Zuck introduce new features that have influenced your usage?

To make sure your relationship with social media doesn't drift back into vampire territory, take time to go back and restate your intention regularly. Why am I here? What need is this platform meeting or not meeting? Take an honest look at how that relationship is going. Is social media working for you or the other way around?

Energy is work. Keep it flowing in the direction that takes you where *you* want to go. Because the only place the Meta-verse wants you to go is to the next ad, and the next ad, and the next ad. And you didn't get sober to buy cube pillows and Moon Juice.

THE ENERGY OF US: NAVIGATING THE WORLD

Sometimes it feels like if we could simply focus on ourselves and the people around us, we might just succeed at managing our lives. But then the rest of the world does something obnoxious to remind us that it is there. This may feel overwhelming in the moment, but it is a good thing. We need community around us, including communities we might not yet know we're a part of. The world is an expansive and magical place, and the more we can learn to connect to that energy and magic, the more generous we can become and the greater freedom we will experience.

Unfortunately, many of the reminders we receive of the world around us have more to do with capitalism than mutual, magical relationships. But if we want to free our spirits and our energy to support our communities, we must learn to manage the unpleasant demands of life as well. The practices in this section offer suggestions for how to tackle areas of life that we may have neglected while drinking or using. It concludes with a call to learn how substance use disorders intersect with larger social issues and how your sobriety can make you an agent of change.

CHAPTER 12

RECOVERING YOUR HOME

"The question of what you want to own is actually the question of how you want to live your life."

— MARIE KONDO

There was always that tube of concealer.

It was there for me when the rings under my eyes betrayed long nights of drinking. When my skin would break out from eating pizza and bar food too many days in a row. When I needed to look perky and engaged instead of pale and hellishly hungover.

Over the years, the brand changed, but that tube was always there.

After I quit drinking, my skin wasn't perfect, but I no longer felt that my face needed to be concealed. I even kicked my decades-long habit of closely examining my skin in the mirror, picking at imperfections and obsessing over new wrinkles and blotches. Giving that up wasn't a conscious choice. I simply didn't have the same compulsion to focus on my flaws.

But whenever I came across the concealer in my makeup bag, a familiar, uneasy feeling would unwind itself in my belly. Seeing that tube reminded me of blurry mornings and shaky hands. At one point, the concealer had been a co-conspirator who helped me hide my secrets and pass as a functioning adult. Now, it felt like an unwelcome visitor from my past.

So, I threw it away. The *thunk* it made when it landed in the garbage was so satisfying that I decided to throw all the rest of my pre-sobriety makeup away, too. Then I scrubbed my whole bathroom, lit some candles, and took a bath. That week, I bought a little plant for my vanity. I even got a new shower mat.

This was early in my energy work journey, so I didn't understand that what I was doing instinctively was space clearing.

Bathrooms held a lot of drinking energy for me. For better or for worse, drunk people spend a lot of time in the bathroom.

Women's rooms at bars and concerts inspire friends and strangers alike to drunkenly bond and lift one another up–something I honestly miss.

I do *not* miss sitting on the toilet to gauge my intoxication level. (Spinning? Tipping over? Able to easily stand back up? How much more can I get away with before they'll stop serving me?) Yikes, that's hard to see written out in black and white.

And then there were nights when too much booze and too little food found me face-down in the toilet. *Yuck.*

The bathroom where I did my space clearing had a skylight that let the morning sun pour in and highlighted evidence of the damage I was doing to myself. Much concealer was applied in that room.

Those memories are painful, but I've made peace with them. Transforming my bathroom was a big part of finding that peace.

Getting ready is no longer a reckoning. It's an opportunity to high-five myself for staying sober another day in a space clear of chaotic, regretful energy. I will never, ever take for granted the bliss of a morning unhaunted by the specter of last night's overindulgence.

Shortly after I ditched the concealer, I came across a book called *Recovering the Home* that shed some light on why the simple act of cleaning out my bathroom felt so huge. Most of what I'm going to share with you in this chapter comes from *Recovering the Home* and from multiple conversations I've had with the author, Jocellyn Snyder (neé Harvey), who has since become a friend (and gave me permission to write about her system, because she's the best!).

 *To listen to my interview with Jocellyn on the Feminist Hotdog podcast, visit **bigsoberenergy.com/reader-bonuses**.*

Jocellyn isn't on social media anymore, but when she was, the photographs of her home always looked like an "after" photo in a magazine spread about decluttering. Her rooms featured tasteful, neutral furniture and smooth surfaces adorned with well-curated knick-knacks. Jocellyn herself always wore natural-fiber basics that perfectly complemented her surroundings. If you're going to take lifestyle advice from anyone, she's an excellent choice.

Jocellyn told me she decided to write *Recovering the Home* to share her love of decluttering with other sober people and to boost her own confidence as a writer in recovery.

"In my first year of sobriety, I was spending a lot of time at home, and I was looking around and noticing how off-kilter I felt with the things in my home and why I had purchased them," she told me. "At the time, I went through the Marie Kondo book [*The Life-Changing Magic of Tidying Up*], and I really liked it. Then, a few years later, I had a creative itch. I wanted to get back into writing, and I thought, 'How can I bring together my love of writing, my love of talking about recovery, and also my love and knack for being able to declutter and organize?'"

In her book, Jocellyn shares a harrowing story about a jacket she'd once loved but ultimately decided to part with. The jacket was still in beautiful condition, but it carried memories of a particularly awful night when she'd embarrassed herself in front of co-workers, then gone to the grocery store in a blackout and "woken up" at the checkout buying $100 worth of groceries she couldn't afford.

"The jacket just did not feel good anymore, even though it was an aesthetically appealing jacket," she explained. So, off to the thrift store it went. Also gone, among other things, were her bar cart, over-the-top party clothes, and the collection of Advil bottles she used to keep next to her bed.

"[I]n the rooms of AA, they talk about your inside and your outside not matching each other, and just that uncomfortable feeling," Jocellyn reflected. "And as I started to declutter, I was able to have my home and my belongings match what I felt on the inside."

The system Jocellyn recommends in her book is pretty intense, but I've included it here because a) I've tried it and it's effective and b) space clearing for people in recovery isn't adequately addressed in other "get organized" guides. Recovering your home is not about becoming a minimalist or a productivity whiz or selling your extra stuff or any of the other reasons people often embark on a decluttering journey. It's about, in Jocellyn's words, "being able to sit in my home, even if it's a messy home, and feel good."

Recovering the Home takes readers through four discrete stages of work:

1. Understanding
2. Aligning
3. Reflecting
4. Personalizing

The full process also involves a set of journaling prompts, which I highly recommend following. Thanks to Jocellyn's generosity, you can download the full text of *Recovering the Home* for free at **bigsoberenergy.com/reader-bonuses,** where you'll find a more detailed description of each step, all the prompts, and a room-by-room decluttering guide.

There is quite a bit of overlap between the four-part Big Sober Energy framework and the four steps of *Recovering the Home.* Since this book aims to support you in learning the intention > meditation > aligned action > integration sequence, I've combined the two frameworks.

Step 1: Understanding (Intention/Meditation)

This first step is all about assessing how you feel and how you want to feel about your space and the items in it. As you focus your intention, visualize opening your closet (or your kitchen or your basement or your car) and liking what you see. Imagine that all the items reflect who you are now and how you want to show up in the world. Then, bring that energy to the rest of the process.

The closet is a great place to start. Jocellyn recommends removing all your clothes, shoes, bags, and accessories, and looking at them honestly to determine your emotional reaction. Be open to whatever might come up. Don't sugarcoat how you're feeling.

My default emotion in this situation is guilt over having wasted money on clothing that I'm now considering giving away. Another big feeling for me is fear of future regret. What if the "perfect" opportunity arises to wear whatever random item has been collecting dust in my closet?

Jocellyn found herself reaching for gratitude when she felt torn or guilty about getting rid of something. After all, wasn't she lucky to have all these things?

"I love gratitude, and that's a big part of a lot of people's recovery," she acknowledged. "But sometimes, you've got to put that aside for a second."

If you struggle to put aside emotions during the Understanding step, bring your meditation practice into play. A short breath meditation will help quiet your mind and bring you into a headspace where you can observe the emotions that arise as you look at your things without having to run away from them.

If the process kicks up something unexpected or you start to panic or spiral, take a break and breathe until you're ready to come back. Jocellyn also recommends informing a supportive friend of your space-clearing mission, so you have someone to reach out to if the piles of stuff start to close in on you, literally or figuratively.

Step 2: Aligning (Aligned Action)

Step two is the step you're probably most familiar with: the physical act of sorting your belongings according to the "keep, give, discard" taxonomy. Here, again, put some bumper rails in place to help you manage stress and keep you centered. Plan in phases, and take breaks. Jocellyn puts a two-hour time limit on work sprints in the alignment phase, regardless of the space she's decluttering.

Items you keep don't necessarily have to "spark joy," as Marie Kondo recommends. But you should have spent enough time with each item to understand if and why you want to keep it and how it fits into your vision for your sober closet, living room, kitchen cupboard, etc.

Jocellyn suggests starting with the "big and necessary" clearing: items that hold overt and covert reminders of your drinking days. In my case, anything wine-stained was an automatic toss. I also ditched anything I'd ever woken up in after a night of going hard and flopping directly into bed.

After removing the worst offenders, move on to tier-two items using the understanding you established in step one to guide you. Use the journal prompts if you decide to go all-in.

Step 3: Reflecting (Integration)

This step is where you lay the groundwork for decisions about the kinds of items you'll bring into your home going forward. Without reflection, it's likely your brain will send a reward signal when you see the same kinds of items you used to reach for while drinking. But once you articulate (and memorialize) your decision not to buy more platform shoes or novelty wine stem tags or whatever, it's much easier to let that impulse pass.

Reflection includes prompts like, "What kinds of items did you tend to keep in your closet? Can you see connections?" and "Were there items you really struggled to part with? If so, why?"

*For the full list of prompts, download Recovering the Home for free at **bigsoberenergy.com/reader-bonuses.***

Don't skip any of the questions in the Reflection step. They could be the difference between keeping your home a relaxing sanctuary or filling it back up with items that dampen your energy.

Step 4: Personalizing (Aligned Action and Integration)

The final step (or rather phase, as it will likely take a while) is to transition your home from a space where things have been removed to a space that fits your energy and your sober life. This is the fun part, where you get to go shopping! (If you find that fun. If not, forget shopping and enjoy the extra space.)

Depending on your circumstances and your budget, shopping might mean a scroll through Etsy, a trip to Costco, or a post on your local buy-nothing Facebook group.

As you think about things you might want or need to add or replace, Jocellyn offers helpful pieces of guidance, specifically tailored for each room in the house. For example, after aligning your closet, she recommends mindful shopping practices, such as trying everything on more than once, saying no to items that are merely "good enough," and keeping the receipts in case you have a change of heart.

Don't overextend yourself financially or energetically in your haste to personalize your home. Personalizing isn't a one-and-done step. Rather, it's a mindset you can cultivate as you think about how you want to live and use your resources. (It pairs well with the concept of "happy money," which you'll read about in Chapter 14!).

Finally, like most things that support recovery, Recovering the Home is a practice you'll want to return to again and again as you learn about your sober self. With every passing day, week, month, and year, you'll crack open new interests, realizations, likes, dislikes, and obsessions you never had time or space for before. You've committed to a sober lifestyle for the long haul. You and your home will evolve together.

You don't have to throw all your stuff away every month, but don't be afraid to shed your skin (or your concealer) as you grow. Over time, you'll become more attuned to your energy. You'll know when the old one starts to feel too tight.

CHAPTER 13

WHAT'S IN THE BOX?

"Start where you are. Use what you have. Do what you can."

— ARTHUR ASHE

One of my favorite writers and thinkers in the recovery space is Holly Whitaker. Holly is the founder of Hip Sobriety and Tempest Sobriety school and author of *Quit Like a Woman*, a groundbreaking book about the intersection of social justice, gender, and Big Alcohol. She's a bonafide powerhouse and one of the most influential voices speaking about sobriety today, but Holly *always* keeps it real in her writing—even when reality isn't very glamorous.

 To listen to my interview with Holly on the Feminist Hotdog podcast, visit **bigsoberenergy.com/reader-bonuses.**

There is no recovery without truth, and the truth is that substance use disorders and sobriety are almost never glamorous. They can be excruciating one day and euphoric the next, but rarely are they smooth and seamless. Nowhere is this more true than in the realm of what early millennial Twitter aptly dubbed "adulting."

Holly recently released an issue of her digital newsletter entitled "The part where you finally open your mail and pay your taxes."

In it, she talks about The Box (capitalization mine) of mail she hadn't opened in a year. She reflected on having been a person who accumulated such a Box when she was drinking, cleared it slowly over the course of the first several years of sobriety, and then found herself once again drowning in unopened envelopes after surviving 12 months marked by a series of emotional blows and personal setbacks (my interpretation, she might describe her experience of those months differently).

Reading about The Box didn't trigger me, exactly, but it did unsettle me. It brought back some pretty terrible memories about missed events, appointments, and deadlines, not to mention a decade's worth of dire financial situations that could have been avoided if I had simply bothered to address them.

But it also brought back a sense of outrage that I felt strongly about then and still identify with today. Because most of the shit in The Box I accumulated wasn't about me or my well-being or my community or my contribution to the world. It was almost all notices about the various systems I was failing to function within. Student loans. Traffic tickets. Medical bills. Taxes. Name any giant bureaucratic machine: I had somehow run afoul of it.

You'll read a sampling of my financial horror stories in the next chapter, but I think it's important to say here that so much of how we define "having our shit together" is about our relationship to money.

Yes, part of the reason I was so bad at keeping my life in order was because drinking took up way too much headspace and contributed to a chaotic lifestyle that in no way supported responsible habits. But part of it was that I was pissed that my worth as an adult seemed to be tied almost exclusively to how well I could navigate what felt like an endless set of tests set up by corporate, capitalist actors who benefited from my failure.

I was (and am) a relatively well-resourced and well-educated white woman—a winner in the privilege lottery. If I couldn't do it, how the fuck was anyone with less privilege and resources supposed to do it? The consequences of a Black woman getting pulled over for having expired tags are incomparable to what would likely happen to me. And why should any of us try to fit into this oppressive, inequitable, cold, inhuman system anyway?

Adding to my resistance was the fact that popular rhetoric about "responsibility" (a favorite topic in self-development crowds) repackages some version of the idea that we, as individuals, are both the cause and the solution of all our own problems. Similar to most manifestation talk, there is almost never any acknowledgment of systemic oppression. Even before I knew how to articulate this, it bothered me.

But while my critique may have been ideologically sound, it didn't apply in my case because I had, in fact, caused most of my own adulting problems. *Damn it.*

What's more, my one-woman anti-establishment crusade wasn't helping anyone, including people more oppressed than I was, and it certainly wasn't tearing down any unjust systems. It only hurt me and weakened my ability to advance my life to a place where I could become an agent of change or tend to the areas of my life that *were* important to me.

I spent so much energy trying to put out fires (like getting boots off my car or unfreezing my student account so I could print out my papers for class) that I rarely, for example, attended meetings of the graduate teaching assistants' union I belonged to or showed up for my volunteer gig reading to kids at a local elementary school. I wasn't present for myself or my community.

Lost invitations meant I showed up late on friends' wedding days.

Missed graduation correspondence from the university resulted in my name being misspelled on my diploma.

I once left a box of fruit my mom had sent at the post office for three weeks after I got the package slip in the mail. When I finally bothered to pick them up, the oranges were deflated and black with mold.

All that to say, The Box is unpleasantly familiar. It's more than simply evidence of our neglect. In many ways, it's a metaphor for everything we refuse to look at while we're drinking and using. Like the story about Pandora, The Box held demons I never wanted to face.

But if there is no recovery without truth, then at some point we have to take an honest assessment of where we've fallen behind and hurt ourselves in the process. Unlike Pandora, opening The Box can lead to healing and even small-scale liberation. It offers an opportunity to reclaim our time. It offers us evidence of energy well spent.

INTENTION

When it comes to taking care of the pesky details of life, resistance often comes in two forms. One, we don't want to do it because it annoys, bores, or distracts us from something we'd rather be doing. And two, we don't want to do it because we've let it go for so long—the literal or metaphorical Box has gotten so full—that even thinking about dealing with it induces a panic attack.

This is where intention-setting can be a lifesaver.

If your intention is focused on organizing your whole life and resolving every outstanding issue that's lurking in your unopened mail, the likelihood that you'll make and maintain progress is basically zilch.

But if you focus instead on setting micro-goals and spending your energy in small, manageable chunks, The Box starts to feel less like a punishment. Instead, it becomes a way to practice the experience of making gradual, incremental progress—the way most sustainable, self-directed life changes happen. Micro-goals reinforce for our conscious *and* our subconscious minds how small, daily actions can prevent anxiety and save us so much energy over time.

The second big intention-setting lesson I want to impress upon you is this: Taking care of your shit is going to look different for everybody.

Not everybody has The Box. For you, getting your life together might look like creating a routine, establishing medical care, learning to be more punctual, or pursuing an educational opportunity.

When I interviewed one of my favorite fellow podcasters, Cynthia Wright (host of *Getting Your Shit Together*—highly recommended), she told me that, for her, getting her shit together started with taking therapy seriously for the first time, which led to pretty much everything else she accomplished in sobriety. Your adulting intention will be unique to you.

 To listen to my interview with Cynthia on the Feminist Hotdog podcast, visit **bigsoberenergy.com/reader-bonuses.**

Maybe you don't care about your unopened mail, and that's fine. Your life stressors may go way beyond anything you currently have control over; I get that, too. But you owe it to yourself to identify—and eventually face—those neglected life details that you *do* have control over, the ones that troll your mind, robbing you of your energy and your joy.

Life is stressful enough without the stress we cause ourselves. Be like Cynthia, and take the task of removing that stress seriously. Your future self will thank you.

MEDITATION

Have you ever moved across the country? The amount of adulting a transition like that requires is bananas. Renting vans, packing, turning utilities on and off, changing your address, getting a new driver's license, finding a new bank/gym/doctor, enrolling kids in new schools—it's a fucking nightmare. Anyone who tells you it isn't is either a masochist or a liar.

I recently had the displeasure of moving from the East Coast to the West Coast of the United States. Even though I was excited about the destination of the move, the experience of juggling so many logistics at one time ground me down to a nub. Coherence meditation is *the* practice that kept me alive and relatively sane. (To be transparent, I also went back on antidepressants during this time and could not be happier about that decision).

Put simply, Coherence meditation allows you to align your heart and mind. The theory is that by focusing on and generating the feeling you want in your body, you will invite more of that feeling into your life.

If you can, do this meditation in the morning before the reality of the day fully sets in. Even if you are trying to be better at life, DO NOT CHECK YOUR EMAIL FIRST THING IN THE MORNING. Use this liminal time when your brain is more open to reduce your stress, not add to it.

In the context of taking care of your shit, a Coherence meditation goes like this.

- Take a few minutes to listen to your breath and practice observing and letting go of your thoughts.

- Then, let yourself visualize a future where whatever is waiting for you in The Box or side-eyeing you from your to-do list is taken care of. Not only is it taken care of, but your whole life feels seamless and orderly. In this reality, you are *your* ideal version of responsible and organized. (Again, this will be different for everyone and does not have to conform to any external standard.)

- Give yourself permission to live in that reality for several minutes. What does it look like, taste like, smell like, sound like, *feel* like? Allow yourself to exist in the state of being free from preventable stress. Experience it at a cellular level.

Whether or not you believe in the energetic magnetism of a Coherence practice, it will work—or at least help. Why? Because, when we label ourselves and our lives as chaotic and messy, we make it harder to align our energy and our actions with calm and order. And it makes sense that we might gravitate toward chaos, especially if we've been drunkenly flying by the seat of our pants for a few years. Chaos can be comforting.

This visualization helps us rewrite stories that might be keeping us stuck in chaos by associating calm, comfort, and relaxation with a vision of life where mail is opened, appointments are made and kept, and applications are submitted on time. It's never going to be "perfect" because perfection is a construct that doesn't exist (and thus striving for perfectionism is a road to self-defeat). But meditating on a future where you've achieved *your* ideal level of life-taken-care-ed-ness can empower you to see and *feel* your way forward.

This vision will be harder to achieve for some people than for others based on income, time, neurodivergence, and what was modeled for them at home, among other factors. But everyone has the capability to decide what their version of having their shit together looks like and the freedom to visualize it, and that is a powerful place to begin.

ALIGNED ACTION

Some of my favorite suggestions for keeping life at least semi-on-the-rails were gifted to me by friends with ADD and ADHD. I'm wary of making too broad of a statement here, but in my experience, folks who are neurodivergent in this way have found some of the most creative and effective ways to consistently accomplish the mundane tasks that life demands, despite having brains that would rather be finding the next and the next and the next thing to be excited or curious about.

I mentioned Amelia Jones in Chapter 7, Body and Soul. Amelia is a neurodivergent, trans alchemist and witch who works in several modalities related to voice healing, plant medicine, and embodiment. They are the person who first introduced me to EFT and one of my greatest inspirations when it comes to finding ways to manage mundane tasks so they don't wind up in The Box.

Amelia described having ADD as, "time and space existing in a non-linear plane of inspiration." For them, what may appear to be chaos, lack of structure, or schedule, is really another way of existing and creating unique, individual patterns fueled by inspiration and wonder.

"This sounds lovely, until you force in patriarchal-capitalist-colonialist structures that are more concerned with production than the art of creating," they told me. "How we define ADD emerges from these structures and sadly, only gets acknowledged when things go 'wrong.'"

For Amelia, having ADD often means doing things that seem like a waste of time but are, in fact, listening to and feeding their body and mind in ways that lead to some pretty magical places.

Unfortunately, the rest of the world remains on a schedule that often feels out of sync with their unique rhythm. Their solution to surviving in the material world without sacrificing their inner world?

Robots.

"I call all technology 'robots' and 'tech faeries,'" Amelia explained to me. "I view them as my friends who help me navigate the world."

By assigning the adulting to the robots and faeries, Amelia is able to enjoy the fantastic voyage that their ADD mind takes them on without constantly worrying that they've forgotten something.

They may not keep to a traditional schedule, but they find the expansiveness to create while still running a business.

They are one of the most disciplined people I know about putting their phone down and getting out in nature.

And they energetically engage in practices like meditation, visualization, intuitive movement, and singing as tools for expressing and feeding their creativity while still staying on task and anchored in time.

"Music is integral to my ability to enjoy 'adulting,'" they told me. "Vibrational medicine is an ally I can always rely on to nourish my nervous system, mind, and emotional self. I could feel like I'm about to have a panic attack, then play a specific song or piece and feel an immense shift in my internal reality."

Whether or not an ADD diagnosis is part of your story, we can all learn so much from Amelia and their wisdom. Here are a few of the suggestions they shared with me to share with you.

1. Find a pretty, user-friendly task app that you will want to open (or apps—you may want one for work, one for budgeting, etc.). Amelia is partial to Structured.

2. If analog is more your thing, invest in a planner that is designed to capture whole-life tasks and details. I'm partial to the Panda planner and the Full Focus planner, but there are many good ones out there.

3. Establish an energetic relationship with the app or planner. Make it your ally or your employee or your helpful assistant robot or whatever works for you. The point is, don't think of interacting with the app or planner as another thing you have to do. You are assigning it to do work for you.

4. Designate specific times of the day and week for adulting, and then put your phone away as much as possible. (See also Chapter 11, Make Social Media Work for You.) Phones like to make us believe we are being productive by staring at them, but you and I both know that 85 percent of the time we have our phones in our hands, we're not doing anything that serves us or our recoveries.

5. If the app you use isn't the kind that beeps or blorps to let you know it's time to move from one task to another or go to your dentist appointment or get dressed for your sister's wedding, set those alarms yourself. If we can disassociate alarms from the horrors of waking up hungover on a workday, those little bells or whistles can be life-giving tools.

6. Again, you can go analog with this. Kitchen timers and Casio watches beep as loudly as phones.

7. Automate and outsource as much as you can. Look for ways to inexpensively offload the tasks you don't want to have to do or keep track of and let those uninteresting-but-necessary details hum along in the background while you live your actual life.

8. Make sure to schedule time to move and breathe and do all the things you are learning in this book! They may not immediately seem "productive," but finding that mental space and energetic balance will positively affect your ability to take care of your shit.

Experiment, rinse, and repeat until you find the combination of tools and strategies that work for you. Even if it takes a while, resist the urge to call yourself hopeless or lazy or to beat yourself up for being disorganized. The cognitive load required to function in modern society is more than most people can handle. The cracks may not show in the same ways for everyone, but they are there. Be kind to yourself, and work with your mind, not against it.

As Amelia says, "Having what is defined as ADD is brilliant, in my opinion. The most inspiring, resilient people I've met learn how to tap into their unique rhythms, and it's really beautiful to witness."

INTEGRATION

Programming the robots and clearing The Box are huge accomplishments. But how can we make meaning of those experiences and help ourselves maintain our adulting habits so we don't wind up pushing the same boulder up the same hill?

We know from our friend neuroscience that overcoming addiction is almost always a function of rewiring our reward systems, offering our brains an alternative to toxic substances when we experience a trigger. If feeling like a loser who doesn't open your mail is a trigger for you, I encourage you to start rewarding the fuck out of yourself. For everything. All the time.

Open one piece of mail, and listen to your favorite song five times in a row. Open ten pieces of mail, and order a pizza for dinner.

Throw yourself a party every time you cross something off your To Do list. Make it fun! Color, skip, play video games. The more childish the activity, the better (to balance out all the grown-up crap).

Keep your marked-up to-do list and look at it whenever you need a boost. You can even rename it: the *I Did It!* list.

Changing habits and getting organized is long-term work. Staying motivated is key because being crushed under the weight of your to-do list is an isolating and shameful experience. Leaning on your community is another powerful way to integrate that experience and put yourself in the path of people who have gone through the same thing.

Maybe you have a friend who struggles with the same kinds of tasks and you can make regular "taking care of business" dates. Opening mail is more fun with friends! Or, perhaps they like to clean, and you like to balance checkbooks, so you can trade adulting labor while you learn more about each other. If your friend is also sober, these times of mutual support can become powerful and cherished moments of your respective recovery journeys.

The value of these shared moments is another bit of wisdom I took away from my interview with Cynthia Wright when she described making *Getting Your Shit Together* as a form of therapy. Specifically, she noted that hearing from listeners and guests about the different ways they got *their* shit together helped her think more expansively about her life and recovery.

> *It's been such a gift for me, meeting different types of people, different ways of approaching things. I've learned as much from other people that have been on my show than [from] anything.... It's been so helpful and beneficial for me to tap in and connect with people in a way that's not about feeling guilty or shameful, but just being honest about where we are, whether it's a great place or whether it's a very shitty, messy place.*

The raw honesty of *Getting Your Shit Together* is like a balm for me as a listener, because every episode normalizes for me that there is no end-point to being a "recovered" adult. Nothing about this experience is linear. People level up and down over and over again in terms of how successfully they handle their lives—and that's okay.

It's more than okay. It's human. And nakedly embracing humanity—in all its glory and shittiness and boxes of unopened mail—is what recovery is all about.

CHAPTER 14

BANISH THE MONEY MONSTER

"About the only thing we can imagine is catastrophe."

— DAVID GRAEBER

When I was in my drinking heyday, my financial management strategy boiled down to three words: swipe and pray.

Despite having an okay job and a decent amount of training on how not to abuse and neglect my bank account, I never knew how much money I had, how much I owed, or when my bills were due. If I maxed out my only usable credit card, I simply opened a new one. I shudder to think how many thousands of dollars banks have made off my use of their overdraft "protection" services. I gambled hard on the fact that bars wouldn't run my card until after I'd had my fill of vodka gimlets. And you know when you buy booze on airplanes and the flight attendant runs your card through a hand-held credit card machine? Those machines don't connect until touchdown. I counted on that, too.

Even worse, I borrowed money like the world was ending—and not only on credit cards. A semester's worth of student loan money disappeared within weeks. I was on a first-name basis with the woman who staffed the payday loan counter. (I even knew the date of her wedding—cringe). When unexpected expenses hit, I invariably hit up my more fiscally stable friends for loans rather than sorting out the situation myself. Looking back, I'm horrified that I was that friend. At the time, though, it was the only way to maintain what I perceived as a non-negotiable lifestyle of partying and bar hopping.

I told myself many stories about why I handled money the way I did (or didn't): I was a mooch, an irresponsible degenerate, a financial loser who was too dumb to balance my checking account.

Under closer scrutiny, however, those stories didn't hold up. Because once alcohol was no longer running the show, about 75 percent of my money issues disappeared.

I didn't take a class or commit to a debt-reduction program or download a special app that gave me an electric shock when I was about to overdraft my account. I was simply no longer living under the spell of the context-dependent memory cycle.

You'll remember our old friend the context-dependent memory cycle from Chapter 5. It turns out the "trigger > behavior > reward" pattern applies to more than drinking and using drugs. It applies to *any* behavior that gives our brains a dopamine bath, even if that behavior is harmful to us—like spending compulsively or avoiding money issues.

Say, for example, I'm walking down the street feeling a bit down about myself, and I pass a shop with a pair of shiny gold shoes in the window. My brain might say to me, "You would feel so much better walking down the street in those dope shoes!" and I would have to agree.

Out comes the AmEx, regardless of how much I can afford to spend on shoes at that moment (or on gold shoes, ever). And, for a few hours or maybe even a few days, looking down at my glittery feet *does* make me feel better.

But then, the thrill of the catch begins to fade. And then the credit card bill arrives. *Damn.*

The arrival of the bill is another trigger. I didn't know the balance was that high. Ugh. Thinking about my overspending makes me feel bad; making a plan to deal with this bill seems hard and stressful. What does *not* seem hard is folding up the bill and sticking it in a drawer. That's better. I put that situation out of my mind and focus on something else. My stress subsides—for now. Sweet, sweet ignorance, a balm for the brain!

To translate this pattern into energy terms, the energy that ruled my money life mirrored the energy that ruled my drinking life: frantic, compulsive, obsessed with my immediate comfort, and allergic to thinking about my long-term health. This made it feel easy and natural to live on the edge of bankruptcy and blow off my money woes because I already lived my life snugly curled up in a neural pathway carved out by the trigger>>behavior>>reward cycle. It was uncomfortable, but it was familiar.

The good news is that rehabilitating my toxic drinking habits drastically improved my money life. I breathe a lot easier now when I open my credit card bills. When I enter my pin into an ATM, I no longer silently beg it to "make the money sound!" My debt-to-income ratio has finally nudged my credit score into the "good" zone.

Quitting drinking wasn't a silver bullet; I still had to reorient my relationship with money, and it's a road I'm still traveling. But recognizing and shifting the energy I brought to that relationship created some of the most tangible and empowering improvements to my life in recovery. It's why I'm so passionate about teaching money energy practices.

If we don't recover our financial lives, two things happen. One, our brains remain in the comfort zone of avoidance and instant gratification. And two, we continue to believe stories about ourselves that make us feel weak and unworthy.

Neither of these things is safe for people with substance use disorder.

INTENTION

I am not a financial advisor, and my intention is not to give you a financial rehabilitation plan. I'm not even going to tell you to create a budget or a debt reduction schedule. Yes, those things are important, but if you're anything like me, they're the equivalent of being advised to run a marathon when you can barely walk to the corner. Diving directly into responsible adult mode is a setup for failure if your money brain stopped developing in your early twenties.

Before you can catch up, you must examine how you feel about money and why. Then, get clear about your intention to establish a new energetic relationship with currency. This commitment is critical to changing your habits and growing your wealth.

Yes, your *wealth*—the wealth you are 100 percent entitled to, even if you drank your face off and did stupid shit for too many years. That wealth.

MEDITATION

Once you have set your intention, take some time to explore the origins of your money stories. I like to do this in two ways: automatic writing and affirmations. Both are best accomplished after a meditation session.

Begin with a 10-minute vipassana (breath) meditation, and permit yourself to notice your thoughts without trying to control them. Focus on breathing; if your mind wanders, simply bring your attention back to your inhales and exhales.

Immediately after your meditation, ask yourself the following questions:

What is my earliest memory of learning about money?

What messages did I hear growing up about money? Where/from whom did I hear them?

When my family discussed money, I noticed _____, and I felt like _____.

Do I consider myself to be "good" or "bad" with money?

Who do I know in my life who "has money"? How do I feel about them?

What do I believe about people living in poverty?

What do I believe about people living with wealth?

Don't think about the answers; let your pen flow over the paper and record the first words that come to your mind.

Finally, take a look at what you wrote, and pick one money story you would like to focus on first. This story will become the basis for an affirmation that can help shift your limiting beliefs and the corresponding energy.

If you realize that you consider yourself to be "bad" with money, for example, your affirmation might be something like, "I have the skills and the fortitude to learn everything I need to know about finances."

If your meditation revealed that you feel negative emotions about people with wealth, you could try something like, "The more money I have, the more generous I can afford to be."

For more about how to write and integrate affirmations into your life, see Chapter 6.

ALIGNED ACTION

Face the Money Monster

Part of the reason I never wanted to know how much was in my bank account or my total credit card debt is that, on the rare occasions I mustered up the courage to look, the reality was worse than my fears. I'm not saying that to discourage you, only to reinforce that avoiding the situation absolutely makes it worse. The monster will never be smaller than it is today, so you might as well look under the bed now.

But here's a secret: Shining a flashlight into the snake pit of your financial situation doesn't mean you have to do anything about it. Energetically, you're making a giant shift just by looking—and then looking again and again.

One of the first and simplest action steps I teach students is to check their bank and credit card account balances every day. Yes, every day. That might seem kind of extreme, but building financial stamina is like building any other muscle: You have to start small enough that getting consistent doesn't fatigue you. Psyching yourself up to check your balance might be all the energy you have to give your financial life on a given day, and that's fine. Think of it as a ritual rather than a chore.

Facing the monster is more than an exercise. Seeing the pluses and minuses in real time, watching where your money goes, when your bills come due, and how much the accrued interest is costing you—all of these data points can transform how you approach your financial decisions. Order takeout or cook the vegetables wilting in your refrigerator? Buy a dress for your cousin's wedding or Rent the Runway?

Again, you don't have to change your behavior if you don't want to—yet. But operating from a place of awarenean empowering experience. Over time, these experiences can begin to change your brain and make you hungry for more empowerment. That hunger can begin to inspire small changes in your money mindset and decision-making—changes you may not even be conscious of until the next time you check your credit score and find it in the green.

Reimagine the Nature of Money

For many years, money was truly monstrous to me—terrifying in its scarcity and its power to make me feel small and stupid. I looked at people who were "good" with money with envy. How did they attract dollars like magnets while I seemed to repel them? It made money seem cruel, like it was personally mocking me.

What changed my mind was a short book by an author named Ken Honda: *Happy Money: The Japanese Art of Making Peace with Your Money*. In this book, Honda argues that money is a harmless, neutral energy, but that, because we live under capitalism, its energy changes depending on how it is spent, hoarded, or moved around.

OK, I may have added the part about capitalism. But it makes sense. In a society where basic needs are only available to those who can pay for them, money reigns supreme and takes up a jumbo-sized amount of space in most of our brains. What we think and how we feel about money influences many of our choices and behaviors, even the ones that aren't explicitly money-related.

If we grew up in a home where money was scarce and caused family conflict, money might feel scary, dangerous, or elusive. If we're in a cold, unloving relationship where money is weaponized or substituted for affection, money might carry a needy, empty energy for us. But consciously changing the energy we project onto money is a tool all of us can use to change these stories. Mastering our money energy gives us more control over our ability to make, keep, give, and spend money with joy and fulfillment rather than anxiety and dread.

Before I go any further, I must point out in the strongest terms that our position in society significantly influences our access to resources and opportunities. There is no doubt that changing money stories and trajectories will be harder for people who experience systemic oppression. Despite what Napoleon Hill would have you believe, the ease with which we can change our incomes is not equally distributed.

But shifting money energy is possible for and available to everyone. It can have tangible, material effects, and these effects can benefit us as we fight unjust and exploitative systems. Working to improve our money stories and situations and working to improve our world are not mutually exclusive. Pursuing money under capitalism is not an endorsement of capitalism—it's survival.

So, if money feels scary and scarce, how do we change that?

The key, says Honda, is to strive to have a flow of *happy* money around us, "money circulated with love, care, and friendship." Happy money is earned through an honest exchange between someone who proudly and joyfully offers a service (or good) to a buyer who willingly and enthusiastically receives it. Happy money grows when we approach life with an open hand, giving what we can afford to those in need with no expectation of being paid back. Happy money flows in and out of our lives when we are learning, growing, seeking, serving, connecting—*living*. When life feels stagnant, or our bank account feels like our enemy, focusing on restarting the flow of happy money can help us return to a place of abundance.

Even earning or spending just a few dollars in this way can make a huge difference!

The concept of Happy Money sparked such an intense *"a-ha!"* moment in me that I felt my brain lighting up. At the height of my drinking (and resulting financial disasters), my money flow and related emotions looked like this:

MONEY IN	
SOURCE	**EMOTION**
Toxic job	Desperation, fear that my soul was disappearing little-by-little each day
Kind friends lending me money	Shame and discomfort for me; annoyance and dwindling respect from them
Predatory lending institutions	More shame and desperation plus a side of bitterness
Credit cards and student loans	Fear that the well would eventually run dry
MONEY OUT	
Bars	Comfort initially, followed by disappointment and self-loathing
Take out	Same as above
Groceries	Optimism that I was preparing to eat healthily, followed by more self-loathing when I threw out soggy bags of rotten produce two weeks later

Massive student loan and credit card payments plus other mounting debts	Disappointment, anger, despair that I would ever see a zero balance in my lifetime
Rent	Resigned but unsettled due to how much income it devoured
Charges on credit cards for travel, concerts, etc.	Excitement and entitlement followed by avoidance and depression
Parking tickets, overdraft fees, late fees	Blind rage

Tally up that emotional ledger, and it's not hard to see that my money flow carried a costly emotional weight. It felt like a swirling drain, pulling me into an inky abyss. It felt like I was drowning.

But, according to Ken Honda, it doesn't have to be this way. Once you identify where your flow is stagnant or why your money feels unhappy (yes, this is a thing!), you can empower yourself to change it. Simply understanding that money carries energy is a huge step. Shifting how you treat money, from whom you accept money, and how generous you are can significantly impact your financial life *and* your emotional life.

Another technique for reimagining money comes from Dr. Kate Tomas. In her work as a spiritual empowerment mentor, she noticed that women and femmes tend to project male energy onto money. Because we live under capitalism and patriarchy, imagining money as male leads many of her clients to develop blocks that interfere with their efforts to gain and maintain wealth—especially if they've experienced trauma at the hands of men. If money equals violence, dominance, manipulation, or shame, why would anyone want to invite that energy into their life?

While entirely understandable, equating money with trauma only disempowers us further by keeping us poor.

The antidote Kate recommends is changing the subconscious narrative by thinking of money as a woman or anyone you do not want to see under the control of oppressors (Kate views gender as fluid, expansive, and non-binary). She explained this so beautifully on an episode of *Feminist Hotdog* that I want to share it here.

> *Even if it's just for the purposes of claiming back power from the oppressors, I'm happy to gender money as female. And then it becomes a totally different story. Getting money, pulling money in, feeling entitled to money becomes something that you're doing for your sister, who is under the control of oppressors.*
>
> *A foundational stone to my teaching is that the solidarity of the oppressed is absolutely central to our liberation, and that there is a very particular type of solidarity between people who are not men and specifically between women.*
>
> *So, when we gender money as another woman, then it becomes very much easier for us to say, 'You know what? You don't get to control that woman. I'm going to help her be free from you.' And by you, I'm talking about the corporations. I'm talking about the cis white men that currently control so much of the money.*

Isn't that *cool*? I fucking love it.

 To listen to my interview with Dr. Kate Tomas on the Feminist Hotdog podcast, visit **bigsoberenergy.com/reader-bonuses.**

With the help of Kate and Ken and a few years of affirmation work, I now feel like money and I are friends. I don't stalk my friend, and I don't ignore her. Our relationship is balanced. I know when my fortunes are up and when they are down, and neither experience changes my sense of self-worth. Sometimes I notice my friend needs more attention than others, and I know I have the capacity to bring our friendship back on course.

And money isn't my only friend. Meditation is my friend. So is listening to music and being in nature. So are my animal and human friends. They all fit together as part of my recipe for well-being.

INTEGRATION

What to do After a Money Meltdown

No matter how happy your money flow or how financially savvy you become, there are always going to be times when unexpected bills or bank account snafus can cause you to lose confidence or make you feel like you're sliding backward. In these moments, how you manage your energy and integrate the experience is as important as the practices described above. I like to break this process down into three Rs: Reset, Reflect, and Refine.

Say you accidentally use your saved debit card information for a large expense you meant to charge on an American Express. The debit goes through, but you overdraft your account. Not only did you incur a fee, but now you have no money to last you until your next payday.

This would be an easy moment to 1) throw up your hands, 2) unleash a string of f-bombs, and 3) maybe even think about taking a drink.

My suggestion? Go ahead and do numbers one and two. Feel your feelings—but put a time limit on it. Give yourself ten minutes to be pissed off, but don't let it go much longer. Set a timer if you have to.

After your fussing time is up, do something to *reset* your body. Your energy is chaotic, and your brain is flooded with adrenaline and cortisol, aka your stress hormones. Get up and walk outside. If you can't walk outside, walk through a doorway to change your immediate environment. Put on your favorite dance song and do some jumping jacks. Gargle warm water. Take a cold shower. Do something physical that will take you out of your headspace. Then, follow it up with a breathing exercise or a short meditation. Doing this will activate the parasympathetic nervous system and help integrate your frantic energy.

Once you feel calmer, take a moment to *reflect* on exactly what happened and how it made you feel. Try to bring a detached mindset to this process. Pretend you are writing a newspaper article. *On March 24, Adrienne van der Valk accidentally used her debit card on file to buy a plane ticket when she had intended to key in a credit card instead. As* *a result, Ms. van der Valk was issued a $35 overdraft fee and will now be eating ramen for the last six days of March. This made her feel very annoyed, frustrated, and ashamed.*

Now ask yourself: What is the worst thing to come out of the situation? How bad is it, really? Six days of ramen is kind of boring but not catastrophic by any measure.

Did anything good come of the situation? Actually, yes. Now the ticket is paid for instead of sitting on the AmEx accruing interest.

And finally: Is there anything you could do to *refine* your actions going forward to prevent this from happening again? In this case, you could remove all credit cards on file with Apple Pay or other electronic wallet services. If credit abuse is the issue, you could relocate your AmEx to the freezer, a clever trick employed by many over-spenders who want to force a waiting period between the trigger (I want to go on a trip!) and the behavior (I'll put the ticket on my AmEx).

Once you've gone through those three steps (four if you count the fussing), say some words of affirmation to yourself, and then let it go. Beating yourself up only robs you of joy and directs your energy toward a bad thing that you didn't want to happen and don't want to have happen again. Deliberately taking yourself through these steps will liberate you from another monster—the shame monster—and remind you that you are a brave human on a difficult journey, and you are doing your best.

Shame is an energy prison. Self-compassion is the key.

CHAPTER 15

CHASING THE GLEAM

"The opposite of addiction is not sobriety.
The opposite of addiction is connection."

— JOHANN HARI

There's a phenomenon I used to experience that I call the "drinker's gleam." It happens when you meet someone and instantly know the two of you are going to get drunk and really *dig in*. It's not sexual (usually), but it feels special and exciting. You and this person are about to become best friends, if only for the night. If you know the gleam, you know.

The problem with the gleam is that it looks shiny, but rarely is it warm and genuine. More often, it's a cold reflection of ourselves. In my experience, it happens when you meet someone who is like you in these three ways:

1. They are energized by alcohol. After your normie friends get tired and pass out, your gleaming friend wants to keep the night going with you.

2. They want to talk about themselves, and you want to talk about yourself. Both of you are willing to validate the hell out of each other in order to be seen as dazzling.

3. Their friends are tired of their bullshit, like your friends are tired of yours. But now you have each other, so you don't need them anymore (at least for now). You can babble the night away with no backstory or bad blood to cloud the atmosphere.

There's nothing inherently wrong with spending the night in the company of someone you just met, bitching about your toxic bosses, or trading tales of sex, drugs, and rock 'n' roll. Where these scenes start to warp is when you decide (at 2:00 am) that this person truly *understands* you and has your best interests at heart.

Don't get me wrong: They may be a perfectly nice person, and you may end up becoming legitimate friends. But at that moment, you know nothing about each other (other than your common love of alcohol– no small thing). This matters little to your prefrontal cortex, which has long since clocked out and gone home. Impulse control has left the building. Time to open the vault of secrets.

It doesn't matter if they're your secrets or someone else's. The rush of false intimacy—sharing information that makes eyebrows raise and jaws fall—is intoxicating all on its own.

And maybe sharing a particular secret comes with an emotional reaction, and this person *gets* it (or at least they shake their head at the appropriate times and say, "Oh my *god!*" a lot). They're *there* for you (aka, they don't nod off or walk away).

Remember, *they* aren't tired of your bullshit. *They* don't know the backstory that paints you not as a victim but as someone who's magnetized to drama like a moth to a flame. *They're* the one you've been looking for—the one who validates you the way you are.

A night of heavy drinking is a lot like a *Choose Your Own Adventure* book. The decision (compulsion might be more accurate) to forego bed, follow the gleam, and spill your guts to a stranger almost never leads to a triumphant ending. For me, the thrill of a drunken bonding session was almost always replaced by a gnawing sense of uneasiness layered on top of my hangover. At the time, I chalked it up to fear I'd be outed, either for an indiscretion I'd shared or for being a bad secret-keeper (more drama—*yay!*). But a few years of sobriety have focused the lens through which I view those experiences.

What I see now is a version of me who was desperate for intimacy and connection. Being someone who can instantly bond with a stranger might seem like an indicator of extroversion or high-functioning social skills, but in my experience, it's a sign of deep loneliness.

Having a substance use disorder is an incredibly isolating experience, even if you're the life of the party. When you have the opportunity to bask in someone's pure, undistilled attention for a few hours, you take it.

So, what are we to make of our attraction to the gleam? Why did I chase these flimsy late-night friendships with the same intensity that I chased the buzz of alcohol?

I drank because I wanted relief from my anxiety (among other stressful emotions). Alcohol was the shortest and easiest path from point A to point B—but it didn't solve anything. That was a design flaw I willingly overlooked. Addressing my anxiety head-on would have taken too much work and too much time. Learning to live with it unmedicated was intolerable. So, alcohol was the answer. Until it wasn't.

Bonding with strangers (or "trauma bonding," as the internet likes to call it) offered many of the same benefits. The false intimacy relieved me of my loneliness and allowed me to feel seen–partially and temporarily. I was lucky in that I had a crew of good friends who stuck by me through my drinking years. But my willingness to be fully seen by them dwindled in proportion to my inability to hide my alcohol use. Trauma bonding was a poor substitute for real connection, but it got me by. Until it didn't.

Here's the thing, though. The more I learn about the relationship between trauma, isolation, and unhealthy coping mechanisms, the less I'm convinced that there's anything all that unique about me or the drinkers and druggers in general. Alcohol isn't the cause of our cravings for false intimacy. Even those of us who are not addicted to alcohol or cigarettes or meth or whatever are looking for love in all the wrong places.

Yes, those of us with substance use disorder might have brains that light up a little brighter once the booze starts flowing. But that's only one point in a constellation of risk factors, and a risk factor you won't find in most surveys (or indexes or longitudinal studies) is living in a society shaped by capitalism, white supremacy, and patriarchy—a society that fundamentally isolates and divides all of us.

INTENTION

Substance use disorder and recovery are not individual experiences because there's no such thing as an individual experience. No person is an island. Everything you think, feel, and do—your energy—touches and has been touched by the people around you, the people who came before you, and the people who will come after you.

There are pieces of you and me and all of us that are divinely unique. But when you were born a human, you joined a species that evolved for interdependence. As much as we might want to believe we're loners, being alone is bad for us.

There's not a whole lot we can do about the inconvenient truth of needing other people. But once we accept this reality, we can use it in many ways to heal ourselves and inspire healing in others.

We can do this by showing up as the most authentic, present, and self-loving version of ourselves in all of our relationships. And we can do this by accepting others for exactly who *they* are and acknowledging our common humanity.

One of the things humanity currently has in common is an uncertain future. Our planet is warming at an alarming rate. Many of us live with political instability and violence, inflation, low wages, and limited access to health care. Our stressors are numerous. We manage them as best we can, and some of our coping mechanisms are harmful.

But one way we can help one another, and ourselves, is by leaning into what we share rather than ranking our coping mechanisms on some arbitrary scale of virtue.

What if, rather than judging ourselves and each other as "better" or "worse" than compulsive porn watchers or crack users or designer drug aficionados or bulimics, we recognized that we are *all* living within systems that, by their very nature, make us sick? What if we looked upon our troubled siblings with compassion and love rather than disgust?

It's tempting to separate ourselves from people we perceive as sicker than we are, but separation is what got us here in the first place. In the words of one of my favorite modern thinkers, john a. powell, breaking down the barriers between us is best achieved through bridging rather than breaking.[24]

MEDITATION

The drinker's gleam was so alluring because of the almost trance-like state two people can fall into when they are buzzing on the same wavelength. You may not spend hours trading secrets in bars any-more, but that doesn't mean you'll never feel that magic again. Allow me to introduce you to your new favorite drug: group meditation.

If anything is guaranteed to convince you that energy is real, it's med-itating in a group. There's a reason most religions encourage people to gather and pray together. Some devotees label the experience as God, others as collective consciousness or universal energy. Whatever you call it, if you've felt it, you know.

It is also the case that collectively focusing our energy can have tan-gible effects. As the witches reading this can attest, we are more powerful together. Large-scale group meditations for healing and peace have been scientifically linked to reductions in violent inci-dents. This is referred to as the Maharishi Effect, as the studies were based on transcendental group meditation under the leadership of Maharishi Mahesh Yogi.[25]

Becoming part of a meditation community online or in person is also incredibly helpful for encouraging consistency, deepening your learn-ing and practice, and building a greater sense of loving connection with the rest of the world.

If you haven't yet found a group to meditate with but still wish to enhance your feelings of community and connection, a metta or loving-kindness meditation is a fantastic alternative.

Metta is a Pali word that roughly translates to friendliness or goodwill. Many origin stories trace the practice back to the Buddha himself, although there is evidence that this concept was explored in earlier Vedic texts.

Unlike vipassana meditation, which asks us to focus our attention on the breath as a means of achieving insight, metta meditation asks us to focus our attention on the sincere wish for happiness, health, safety, and ease—for ourselves and for others.

There are many variations of the practice out there in the world, but a typical metta meditation might go something like this:

Imagine you are speaking to yourself. You may even wish to visualize sitting across from yourself as you speak.

1. Send a tremendous beam of loving energy toward yourself, and as you do this, say these four things to yourself:

> *May you be happy.*
>
> *May you be healthy.*
>
> *May you feel peaceful.*
>
> *May you be loved.*

2. Next, call to mind someone you find easy to love. Once again, call them into your mind's eye, and with a strong, loving energy carrying your voice, say the four things again to your loved one.

3. Then, repeat the same process for the following people:

- Someone you see on a regular basis but don't know well.
- Someone you find difficult, annoying, or challenging to spend time with.

- The people in your neighborhood, city, or town.
- The people in your state.
- The people in your country.
- All living creatures, big and small, the whole world over.

When you're first starting out, it's nice to have a recording or a guide lead you through the practice, but eventually, you will be able to do this for yourself.

Personally, I like to also send loving kindness to everyone in recovery, especially those who might be struggling.

 To listen to a guided metta meditation specifically for people in recovery, visit **bigsoberenergy.com/reader-bonuses.**

Sharing loving kindness with the people around you on a regular basis has some pretty incredible effects. Your empathy grows, your temper subsides, and you feel more connected to others.

Are those changes all in your head? Yes—literally! A 2010 study out of Oxford University offered strong visual evidence that metta meditation physically alters the prefrontal cortex, the part of the brain responsible for decision-making and impulse control.[26]

ALIGNED ACTION

If reading is a big part of your recovery journey like it was mine, this aligned action might make you groan a little. But trust me on this one: Put down books, find a sober community you resonate with, and go all in.

Books are great. I mean...I am telling you all of this in a literal book so, yeah, I think they have a lot to offer! And the stories you read in books do connect you with other people (albeit indirectly), and that can be incredibly helpful, especially in the pre-recovery stage before you've spoken real live mouth-words about the fact that you might kinda sorta have a problem.

We are mammals, and mammals need other mammals to thrive. And, like anything else you learn in life, it's *way* easier to figure out what the fuck you're doing if you can learn with and from other people who are already doing it.

Recovery is hard enough. Don't make it harder by trying to do it alone or by relying on social media or on your partner. Introvert or extrovert, you need this.

Once you've accepted that being a loner-hermit-rugged individualist might not be the lifestyle most conducive to sobriety, what then? It's one thing to know you need a community. How do you go about finding one?

I don't know your life, and I can't ethically answer this question for you. But there are a few things I'd recommend that you keep in mind as you search:

1. Ask a trusted source.

If you are already working with a doctor or social worker or have in the past, ask them for a suggestion. Ditto if you have people in your life who are sober and you feel comfortable asking.

2. Start searching.

If you're doing this 100 percent on your own, you can check out the list of recovery groups at the back of the book. These are options I have either used myself or had recommended to me by people I know and trust.

In almost any community, there will likely be regular AA meetings, which are reliable and free.

And, of course, there's always the University of Google, but blanket searches can be overwhelming and don't necessarily give you the information you need to assess if a group or membership is right for you. If you're already feeling overwhelmed, explore one option at a time.

3. Be willing to "kiss a few toads."

Approach finding a group like finding a therapist or a partner or a lipstick shade that doesn't make your teeth look yellow. Try lots of different options, and by "try" I don't mean go once. Give it a fair shot. If you're not feeling it after three or four gatherings, throw that toad back in the pond.

There are a lot of recovery groups out there, and in early sobriety, having a place to process what is happening to you is invaluable. But don't be afraid to be selective. Just because people will listen and validate you doesn't mean they are your people.

4. Find a space where you can be yourself.

Look for folks who accept your identities and do not require you to suppress who you are in any way. Find a group whose philosophy aligns with your values and supports the full expression of your humanity. If you can make real, genuine community connections part of your daily or weekly schedule, your life just got a lot easier (even if it doesn't feel like it). But if you find yourself hiding or playing small, it means you don't have the space you need to expand into your recovery.

5. Trust your gut.

Recovery communities—even those that exist under the same brand or umbrella—have different flavors because they have different leadership, different members, and function in different cultural settings. None is immune to the exploitation that sometimes occurs when vulnerable people gather together. This is why things often go off the rails when it comes to religion or cults or MLMs or the many intersections of all three. (For a great book on this phenomenon, check out Hey, Hun! by Sober Mom Squad founder Emily Lynn Paulson!)

I'm not saying this to dissuade you but to encourage you to follow your gut. If you run into anyone who tells you not to rely on your gut because you're an addict and you don't know what's good for you, walk away.

6. You don't have to go forever.

While I'm making controversial statements that are probably going to anger some readers, let me go ahead and make another one: You do not have to stay in your recovery community forever. In fact, you may choose an all-in community that's not a recovery community at all.

The community where I've found the greatest validation and support is a spiritual group where most of the members are alcohol-free. That's not a coincidence. Many of the members feel that alcohol disrupts their ability to connect with their guides and focus their energy. The focus is not on sobriety but rather on creating conditions that allow inner work to work. Sobriety is one of those conditions. Daily meditation is another. So is energy mastery.

Maybe your all-in community is a church choir or a running group or an activism circle. It should be a community that does not drink together and where you're comfortable being honest about recovery. Any community can be part of your recovery if you feel safe, seen, supported, and surrounded by the energy you want in your life.

INTEGRATION

Tapping into community isn't just about seeking support for ourselves. It's also about how we show up for other people—including people we don't know.

Truly integrating the concept of community into your recovery means realizing that the pain of substance use disorder hurts all of us and that we all should care about everyone who lives with this pain—even if we don't understand or relate to their lives.

This requires us to expand our definition of community. It means seeking out new stories and common ground. It means choosing compassion and solidarity instead of looking away when other people's journeys feel sad, alarming, or confusing to us.

This approach to integration is particularly important if you are straight, white, and do not currently have a disability. Why? Because people who are queer, trans, Black, brown, or disabled (and all intersections thereof) have already integrated the straight, white, non-disabled recovery experience. It's the version of recovery we see all the time. Think Sandra Bullock's character in *28 Days*, Ron Livingston's *Loudermilk*, and Cynthia Nixon's in *And Just Like That* (Miranda is queer but also wealthy and white).

Most recovery spaces are designed with white comfort and preferences in mind. This isn't necessarily intentional, but it's an outgrowth of the fact that white men founded the early programs from which contemporary recovery evolved. Alcoholics Anonymous, for example, was founded in 1935 by Bill Wilson and Bob Smith, two white Christian men. Their identities and beliefs shaped the 12 steps of AA, and while the program has certainly changed in the intervening century, the fundamental tenets have not.

An example of traditional recovery being inhospitable to people of color is the experience of being redirected for bringing in "outside issues."

Shortly after the summer of 2020, I interviewed writer Jessica Hoppe for *Feminist Hotdog* after reading her *Medium* article, "The First Step to Recovery Is Admitting You Are Not Powerless Over Your Privilege."[27] She shared the story of attending AA meetings in New York City after a Minneapolis police officer murdered George Floyd.

When the people of color in her group shared their grief over Floyd's violent death and the collective trauma so many Black and brown people across the country were feeling, the group leader "redirected" them. The reason given was that current events are political and thus considered "outside issues," interpreted by many AA group leaders to be a deflection and a distraction from the organization's core mission.

Jessica, who is Latina with Black and Indigenous roots, felt blind-sided. How could racism be an "outside issue" when it had such a profound effect on her life and the lives of so many other people in recovery?

---

 *To listen to my interview with Jessica on the Feminist Hotdog podcast, visit **bigsoberenergy.com/reader-bonuses.***

If I had not read Jessica's article, I would not know about her experience. I would not understand why she and many other voices in this space are calling for a reimagining of recovery. I didn't necessarily believe that substance use disorder was the great equalizer, but I naively assumed we would all be treated the same in "the rooms."

We are not.

So, for me, integrating community into my recovery also means recognizing, honoring, and fighting for the larger community of people who struggle with addiction, even if their experiences don't look like mine.

It means opting out of recovery paradigms that gatekeep and police people for sharing their experiences and identities.

It means fighting for an end to the war on drugs.

It means divesting from the way we rank people who drink and use on a hierarchy of worthiness or save-ability.

Absorbing stories about anyone's experience with substance use disorder can result in vicarious trauma. Even trauma you don't experience directly can affect your body. Like with any work that exposes you to other people's energy, it's good to keep your boundaries healthy and to clear your energy regularly. Being in community does not mean you must be a martyr or a saint.

The more attentive we are to our energy, the more fully and authentically we can support and be supported by those we care about. We will no longer feel the need to silence each other. We can stop struggling alone to keep our individual recoveries running unsteadily on parallel tracks, never to meet. We won't need to chase the gleam anymore. We will have each other.

A Note on Individuals and Systems

There's a criticism often leveled against self-development books that goes like this: When we focus on our individual behaviors and relationships, we ignore the harmful systems around us and abdicate responsibility for changing them.

I get that—and I think it overlooks two important things.

One, if we focus only on systems, we deny ourselves access to information that can tangibly improve our lives and well-being. Caring for ourselves and contributing to systemic change should not be mutually exclusive. We are not more virtuous because we neglect ourselves.

Most people are not billionaires and thus not in a position to single hand-edly transform systems. We can all, however, contribute to systemic change if we want to. And we are more effective agents of change when we're rested, centered, and supported.

The second thing this critique overlooks is that systems are made by, of, and for people. Religion is people. Government is people. The prison industrial complex is people.

These systems rely on us internalizing and acting on bias they were built to uphold (by people!). If we don't reckon with our differences, we stand no chance of transcending them. Individuals have a critical role to play in this reckoning.

Change doesn't happen by force. Humans trying to force change upon other humans is generally a doomed enterprise. Force is antithetical to find-ing an ebb and flow of energy that allows us all to connect and thrive.

Change happens within relationships. What allows extremists to leave hate groups? Relationships. What allows teachers to reach students who bully? Relationships. What makes community-based crisis response teams more effective than police? Relationships.

As a society, we should never tolerate unjust or abusive behavior. And, yet, the majority of us do. We see no way to confront the behavior that perpetuates our systems without exhausting ourselves. But individuals hold tremendous power to influence their friends, families, and communities just by speaking and living in integrity. Within relationships, we can sow the seeds of systemic change on a daily basis.

If we want to make the world a more loving and just place, we must think systemically *and* collectively heal ourselves forward (in the words of myisha t hill).[28]

Systemic versus individual is not an either-or proposition. If we fail to understand and bridge the deep disconnects that underpin so many harmful behaviors, how can we work together to repair the systems that broke us apart?

To read more on this topic, visit Appendix A, Writers Who Have Influenced Me.

PART III
THE ROAD AHEAD

CHAPTER 16

QUICK ACTION GUIDES

GETTING STARTED, SOS SITUATIONS, AND GETTING BACK ON THE WAGON

"The progress of tomorrow is the preparation today."

— LAILAH GIFTY AKITA

Whether or not you read this book straight through or skipped around, I want to congratulate you for arriving at this chapter. You wouldn't be here if you weren't committed to *using* this material and harnessing your energy to create a sober life that you love.

There are multiple ways to act on that commitment, and that's what this action guide is all about.

First, we'll look at how to make a Getting Started plan for introducing energy practices into your life in a way that feels sustainable. Like I said in the opening chapters, it would be unrealistic to implement every practice I've shared with you. *I* don't practice everything I've shared with you (at least not all at once). To avoid getting overwhelmed, we'll spend a little time mapping out "what's next?" so you can empower yourself to dive in and begin making energy shifts that align with your vision for your life.

Second, we're going to get real about what to do when you find yourself in an SOS situation. I'm obviously a believer in the power of slow, incremental change and using energy practices on a day-by-day basis. But life is unpredictable. No, it's more than that. Life will, at some point, smack you upside the head and kick you in the shins and steal your milk money, all in quick succession. You'll be hurt, or at the very least confused, and you won't have time to rely on slow, incremental change to help you figure out how to deal.

For those moments, I put together three "Quick Guides" made up of two or three specific practices from the previous chapters, tailored to have the most immediate effect in each specific situation.

Finally, I will share with you my best advice for what to do if you fall off the proverbial wagon and find yourself looking at the bottom of an empty glass, feeling like you've thrown away all your hard work. (Spoiler alert: *You haven't!*)

GETTING STARTED

Creating Your Plan

To create your Getting Started plan, you can use a journal or pen and paper to take notes as you follow along with the steps I lay out here, or you can download a worksheet I created to bring everything together on one page.

 To download the Getting Started worksheet, visit **bigsoberenergy.com/reader-bonuses.**

You may have your own system using calendars or project management software to help you formulate new habits, and if that's the case, definitely use them! The right planning method is the one that you will actually use.

1. Begin by thinking about the distress patterns that show up in your life:

- What are the things you find yourself talking to your friends or your therapist about over and over?

- Where is your life the weakest due to your struggles with substance use disorder?

- What kinds of experiences tend to spike your cravings or at least shake your confidence?

- Are there particular thought patterns or behaviors that you know you need to work on in recovery?

Spend a good five or ten minutes thinking about this. Then, write down four to six chronic stressors that rise to the top for you.

To help you get going, here is a sample *non-exhaustive* list of things that could potentially end up on your list, sorted by life area.

SELF	OTHER PEOPLE	WORLD
Negative self-talk	Tendency to people- please	Difficulty "adulting"
Self-sabotage	Social anxiety	Guilt about privileges I hold
Fear of trying new things	Feeling isolated from friend group	Feeling disconnected from the larger community
Overworking	Family conflict	Professional stagnation
Compulsive shopping	Trouble setting or respecting boundaries	Comparing myself to people I don't know
Feeling unsure about what I want or need	Comparing myself to people I know	Feeling overwhelmed about the state of the world
Replaying past traumas		

In the spirit of transparency, here is my list of current stressors (which is markedly different from the list I would have made when I first got sober).

- Difficulty following through on tasks

- Mood instability

- Imposter syndrome

- Struggling to make friends in a new city

- Feeling overwhelmed about the state of the world

2. Next, take a look at this table and review the benefits associated with the practices in each chapter.

SELF	OTHER PEOPLE	WORLD
Chapter 5: How Do I Feel?*	Chapter 8: Truth Be Told	Chapter 12: Recovering Your Home
Benefits: Self-Awareness, Emotional Regulation	Benefits: Integrity, Stress Reduction, Positive Connection	Benefits: Organization, Emotional Regulation, Stress Reduction, Integrity
Chapter 6: Self-Compassion v. Shame	Chapter 9: What Makes Me Happy?	Chapter 13: What's In the Box?
Benefits: Confidence, Self-Trust, Self-Compassion	Benefits: Emotional Regulation, Self-Awareness	Benefits: Organization, Time Management, Stress Reduction, Confidence, Financial Stability, Integrity
Chapter 7: Body and Soul	Chapter 10: How to Plug an Energy Leak	Chapter 14: Banish the Money Monster
Benefits: Stress Reduction, Confidence, Emotional Regulation, Self-Compassion	Benefits: Positive Connection, Self-Awareness, Time Management, Stress Reduction, Purpose	Benefits: Financial Stability, Confidence, Stress Reduction, Self-Compassion, Integrity
* I recommend that everyone who reads this book includes Chapter 5: How Do I Feel? in their initial plan.	Chapter 11: Happy Place or Hellscape?	Chapter 15: Chasing the Gleam
	Benefits: Time Management, Stress Reduction, Emotional Regulation	Benefits: Positive Connection, Purpose

Based on the stressors you've identified, which benefits do you think would be the most helpful to you? Which do you feel drawn to?

Let's use my list as an example.

- "Difficulty following through on tasks" lines up well with the benefits for Chapter 13, What's In the Box?: organization, time management, stability, stress reduction, and confidence.

- "Mood instability" and "feeling overwhelmed about the state of the world" could align with the benefits for Chapter 9, What Makes Me Happy?: emotional regulation and self-advocacy.

- "Struggling to make new friends" could probably be alleviated by the benefits of Chapter 15, Chasing the Gleam: positive connection, purpose, and fulfillment.

- And having "imposter syndrome" is almost always a symptom of under-developed self-trust—a good reason to re-read Chapter 6, Self-Compassion v. Shame, which offers the benefits of confidence, self-compassion, and self-trust.

This will be an imperfect process! You will have stressors and patterns and people and situations on your list that may not align with the chapters in the book. That's okay—do your best, use your intuition, and trust that you can't screw this up.

3. Once you have identified the chapters you want to focus on, re-read the intention, meditation, practice, and integration steps. Are there any you are already practicing? Which ones feel intimidating to you? Notice how you feel as you read. Where is your energy leading you?

4. Finally, pick up two or three chapters to include in your plan now versus those you'll address later. Some pointers to consider:

Notice which category or categories the chapters you chose fall into (self, others, or world). If they all fall into one category, that's great data for you about where to focus your energy as you start.

If you have selections in each of the three categories, consider picking one chapter from each with the goal of creating more balance in your life.

If you need some additional guidance on which chapter to pick, consider starting with two: one that feels intuitive and easy and one that sparks resistance in you.

And, if this is your first time doing energy work of this type, I want to reiterate the suggestion to include "Ask Yourself 'How Do I Feel?'" in your initial plan. Developing this awareness will help maximize the success of any other practice you choose to engage in.

Narrowing Down Your Priorities

Here's a visual overview of how I might prioritize two of the four stressors on my list, and notes on why.

STEP 1: STRESSOR	STEP 2: BENEFITS	STEP 3: CHAPTER	STEP 4: PUT IT IN MY PLAN NOW OR LATER?	NOTES
Imposter syndrome	*Confidence* *Self-compassion* *Self-trust*	*Chapter 6: Self-Compassion v. Shame*	*LATER*	*Already working on this with therapist*
Mood instability Struggling to make friends in a new city	Emotional regulation Self-advocacy	Chapter 9: What Makes Me Happy?	NOW	Feels the hardest to remember to do
Difficulty following through on tasks	Organization Time management Stability Stress reduction Confidence	Chapter 13: What's In the Box?	NOW	Likely to have quick results
Struggling to make friends in a new city	*Positive connection* *Purpose* *Fulfillment*	*Chapter 15: Chasing the Gleam*	*LATER*	*Not feeling quite ready for this but have started putting out feelers*

Do not let perfectionism sneak into this process! Everything I've included in this book has the potential to benefit you, so if you're taking action, you can't do it wrong. The key is to start small and trust that you will gravitate toward the practices that are right for you.

Recovery is never linear. As time goes by, your stressors and priorities will change, and the tools you need in your toolkit will, too.

I like to think of my recovery as a dashboard on an airplane. When things get bumpy, I turn up the dial on the practices I know have the most immediate effect on my nervous system, my sleep, and my equanimity. When things are a little smoother, I focus on longer-term practices that incrementally build my skills and confidence.

All that to say, you will likely add and subtract and swap energy practices in and out of your plan continuously over time, and that's a good thing. It means you are growing and changing and paying attention to your inner weather forecast.

PUTTING YOUR PLAN INTO ACTION

Now that you have assessed the primary stressors in your recovery and established which practices are likely to offer you the greatest support in mitigating those stressors, it is time to think about how you are going to incorporate these practices into your daily life.

I'll be the first person to acknowledge that this is easier said than done. How do we establish the new behaviors and habits that will help us establish new behaviors and habits?

It may feel impossible if you haven't been successful with these kinds of plans in the past, but I promise you it's not. Once you gain some momentum and begin noticing results, your desire to keep going will become a motivating force all its own. Keep your plan as simple as possible, stay connected to your "why," and follow these three suggestions as you set out to make energy practices part of your routine.

Make the Most of Your Morning

You've read my recovery story, so you know I'm a big believer in using the morning as an opportunity to orient my energy for the day.

There may be good reasons why mornings won't work for you, and I get that. But if you find yourself resisting the idea of a morning practice, I want to ever-so-gently push you to question whether you are putting up barriers that could be creatively navigated. Even if you have kids or a commute or are not a morning person, is there a world in which getting up 15 or 20 minutes earlier might be possible? Or where you could use the commute time for setting an intention or integrating a practice?

If only for a few minutes, try to use that luscious, liminal, post-sleep space to benefit your body and spirit before the rest of the world starts flooding in and wreaking havoc.

Make a Schedule

As annoying as it might sound, I also highly recommend using a calendar or scheduler of some type that allows you to visualize the commitment you've made to yourself and reminds you to keep it. As the obnoxious publisher of my planner reminds me frequently in his marketing emails, "If it doesn't get scheduled, it doesn't get done," and I'm grudgingly inclined to agree.

Of course, not all the practices in this book are things you would do every day, but do your best to at least remind yourself of your intention, complete a meditation, and review the aligned action and integration steps. As time goes on, these daily observations will feel more natural and less time-consuming to complete.

For practices that need attention once a week or a month or a quarter (I'm looking at you, Life Edit), these should go on the calendar, too, but don't forget to add a little fun to the experience. Take yourself out to coffee, run a bath, burn a candle, or pick some flowers. Making energy work into a ritual enhances its power *and* the likelihood that you'll follow through with it (because fun!).

Practice with a Friend

Another thing that makes energy work more fun is friends. If you're part of a sober community, or even if you're not, consider creating an accountability agreement with a buddy and checking off your progress on a shared spreadsheet or text each other a thumbs up when you've completed your daily meditation. Maybe even build in a little social reward to recognize your progress.

SOS SITUATIONS

As a general rule, things that activate your parasympathetic nervous system can be life savers when you find yourself in acute stress for any reason, including cravings, social anxiety, and hearing bad news. The parasympathetic nervous system regulates the "rest and digest" functions in your body, which can help us recover from the immediate effects of a scare or an anxiety spike caused by cravings or other difficult emotional experiences.

The simplest and most accessible way to activate your parasympathetic nervous system is to slow down your breathing. The Integration section of Chapter 5 includes several other techniques such as putting your hand on your heart, taking a walk (in nature if available), playing with a pet, gargling warm water, practicing tai chi or yoga, or getting a massage (if massages are relaxing for you).

I have found that if I assign certain practices to certain types of SOS situations, my brain learns to recognize and respond to what's happening, and I calm down more quickly. In the spirit of making this information as accessible as possible, here are three sets of suggestions you can use to quickly find helpful practices for 1) surviving cravings, 2) dealing with social anxiety, and 3) handling bad news or sudden stress.

Quick Guide for Surviving Cravings

For cravings specifically, these approaches—used independently or in combination—offer a balance of mindfulness, somatic, and pattern-interruption techniques.

1. A fantastic go-to mindfulness strategy for helping ride the craving wave is RAIN, described in detail in Chapter 5.

2. Another suggestion for how to help soothe or distract yourself from cravings is to activate the body, either by using EFT (tapping), singing and laughing, or dancing. Descriptions of all three (and why they're effective) can be found in the Integration section of Chapter 7.

3. A third option for helping cravings subside is to combine a mantra and a visualization. My favorite version of this is to remind myself that "alcohol is attractively packaged poison" while visualizing a skull and crossbones on whatever drink or bottle might have sparked my craving. (Credit for this one goes to Craig Beck and his book *Alcohol Lied to Me*.)

4. You might also remind yourself to "play the tape forward." Then, visualize fast-forwarding through the rest of the night to where you will inevitably end up if you decide to drink *and* to waking up hangover-free the next day if you don't.

Quick Guide for Social Anxiety

There are a few tried-and-true stay-sober tips that belong in everyone's toolkit, like making sure you drive yourself or have access to independent transportation, bringing your own non-alcoholic beverages, and keeping a reliable sober friend on speed dial. Knowing you have made these arrangements for yourself is an energy practice, so don't skip those.

For additional support before and during social situations, take some time to review these practices.

1. As a preventative measure, I suggest getting familiar with the suggestion from Chapter 9 about never saying "yes" in the moment when someone asks you to do something. This will cut down massively on social anxiety because you never have to worry about agreeing to do something you don't want to do. Ditto the Obligation Inventory from the same chapter.

2. Before you head into any social situation, review the energy protection practices in Chapter 10. These include rolling up the window, putting on a mirror suit, and cutting energetic ties with people whose energy lingers after you interact with them.

3. If you're already in a social situation and feel yourself starting to panic, I would again suggest RAIN (Chapter 5) as a highly effective strategy.

4. Remember, you always have the prerogative to leave a situation that is activating you or where someone is disrespecting your boundaries. Remind yourself that no social experience is more important than your well-being!

Quick Guide for Bad News or Sudden Stress

Social obligations usually come with some degree of warning. Bad news does not. For this reason, it is extremely important to create your emergency preparedness kit for when life pulls the rug out from under you.

1. Bookmark an anxiety-reducing meditation on Insight Timer, YouTube, or another platform of your choice. Ideally, use this meditation regularly so your brain identifies the guide's voice with the experience of calming down.

2. Do not face bad news alone. Lean on your community. Even if you don't feel like processing what is happening, attend a meeting or call your therapist if either of those options is in your recovery toolkit. At the very least, reach out to a supportive friend. Ideally, ask someone who knows you are sober to stay with you temporarily while you find your footing.

3. Remain as present as possible. Resist the urge to agonize over the past or project what the bad news means about your future. When you are in crisis, your only job is to feed yourself, drink water, stay sober, and sleep. Anything more will tax you and make it harder to navigate your healing.

4. In all three cases, be sure to integrate your experience before too much time passes. This could be achieved through a somatic practice like yoga, tapping, or walking meditation. You might also choose journaling, talking to a therapist, or writing a "keep, change, throw away" list. In any case, take time to reflect on how you handled the situation and how you would choose to handle it if it arose again in the future.

WHAT TO DO IF YOU FALL OFF THE WAGON

Learning to live without alcohol is a process that almost always involves trial and error. It is extremely rare for people to successfully quit drinking the first time they try. Most people who experience substance use disorder grieve the loss of their relationship with their drug of choice for quite a while. Like with any unhealthy relationship, that grief can become so overwhelming that we decide to "try again," or enough time passes that we forget what was so bad about the situation. You may have fought hard to extract yourself from alcohol's grasp, but there could still come a time when the fight no longer feels worth it, and you have a slip.

As you already know, I don't believe that a single drink or night of drinking means you've erased the progress of your whole sober journey thus far. Don't give a slip-up more power than it deserves. Instead, use it to your advantage.

Immediate Action

1. Do everything I suggest in the Quick Guide for Bad News or Sudden High Stress. Meditate, reach out to your therapist, sponsor, or friend, and remain as present as possible.

2. It will be tempting to catastrophize or even give up and go on a bender. Don't do it. Put one foot in front of the other, then do it again, and do it again. Remember that your anxiety will likely be exacerbated by the addition of alcohol to your system, so what you are feeling is in large part physiological. You will feel much better in a day or two.

Over the Next Few Days

3. Follow whatever advice your therapist or sponsor gives you, even if you don't want to. Part of trusting yourself is trusting that you chose the right people to be on your support team for moments exactly like this.

4. Once you are feeling a bit more stable and out of immediate danger of throwing in the recovery towel, ask yourself how you were feeling leading up to the slip.

   Were there things you normally do that you had stopped doing or vice versa?

Was there a particular person or experience that stressed you or reminded you of the good times gone by? Make an honest assessment of the circumstances surrounding the event.

In the Following Weeks

5. After you've stabilized and are out of immediate danger, revisit the Getting Started process outlined earlier in this chapter (although, in this case, you'll be creating a "Getting Back On Track" or "Keep Going" plan).

   Use the data points you identified in your honest assessment (step 4 above) to guide you in selecting the chapters and practices you will add to your routine.

Allow yourself to get creative, feel some relief, and even have some fun with this process. Remember, this is *your* recovery. Your plan for getting back on the wagon won't look the same as everyone else's.

For example, if you were a physically addicted drinker and having a slip triggered you severely, you may want to spend some time in a therapeutic environment or another place where you know alcohol will not be not available to you.

If you feel devastated by your slip-up, pump up the self-care, self-trust, and self-compassion work.

But if you're not severely triggered or devastated, you don't have to pretend that you are. Slip-ups happen to almost everyone. How you integrate the experience will have a major influence on how you manage the situation the next time you are tempted to hop off the wagon for a night.

You have done the work, and you have the tools you need. Now it's time to remember to use them.

CHAPTER 17

LOOK TO THE FUTURE, BUT DON'T LIVE THERE

"The aim is to balance the terror of being alive with the wonder of being alive."

— CARLOS CASTANEDA

As much trouble as I had figuring out how to start this book, knowing how to end it is equally difficult. There's so much to say about the gifts, struggles, and complexities of recovery and how we can use our energy and love for one another to make it expansive, liberatory, and joyful.

My hope is that finishing this book marks some kind of new beginning for you, whether it's a shift that strengthens your confidence, deepens your fulfillment, enhances your power, or all three.

No one knows what a new beginning might bring or what the future holds, and that's okay. Even before I knew it as a recovery mantra, I understood the wisdom—the comfort, even—of taking life one day at a time.

I'm someone who can get lost in a dream world dominated by fantasies of what could be. I catch myself straining toward a different reality. I have to remind myself of the wisdom of Henepola Gunaratana, that the only guarantee is change. I don't want to live my life running the "perpetual treadmill race to nowhere."

But I do believe there's healing to be found in the future if we can feel our way there—intuitively, gently, and intentionally.

I love to connect with my future self in meditations. I've learned so much and felt so much comfort from her.

I know from experience that envisioning my desired future empowers me and helps me decide how to manage my energy in the current moment.

And, now that I'm sober, thinking about the future fills my present with hope and excitement—not because I'm waiting for a particular thing to happen, but because I realize the gifts of sobriety are endlessly surprising and unknowable.

So, how can we balance these two seemingly conflicting ideas? Is it possible to live in the present moment *and* use the power of our energy to shape the future?

Here is the philosophy I've adopted to help me manage this tension: Look to the future, but don't live there.

Remaining grounded in the now *is* enormously beneficial to us, not only as a tool for navigating cravings, but as a way to support overall happiness. However, if we don't find ways to balance our consciousness of *now* with our consciousness of *later*, we may wind up limiting our potential or boxing ourselves in when expansion would serve us better.

Take the money stories I shared with you in Chapter 14. If I had never thought about the future and lived purely in the moment all the time, it would have been incredibly difficult for me to change my spending habits, especially when it came to credit.

Or take my dear friend Erin who, in the early days of sobriety, suffered from liver disease and felt completely overwhelmed by the knowledge that she was at the end of her drinking days. One of the things that got her through those shaky weeks was planning things to look forward to—specifically tacos and dancing.

We *can* learn to be mindful and still plan for a future we'll enjoy. The key is managing our attachment to the plan and its outcomes.

Get excited about tacos and dancing and improved credit scores or even bigger hopes and dreams. Just don't get so attached to them that your happiness lives or dies by how or when they manifest.

In the words of one of my favorite meditation teachers, Saqib Rizvi, "The best way to ensure that only the best outcome for you is manifested is to place your trust in the universe by surrendering the control of how, in what form, and when that manifestation occurs."[29]

I'm not much of an "everything happens for a reason, the universe has a plan for you" person. But I agree with the wisdom that sometimes the things we think we want won't make us happy. And I believe I owe my sobriety and subsequent changes in my life to the beauty of embracing surrender—not as defeat, but as relief and release and willingness to try another way when the map I was following had long ago disintegrated in my hands.

Allowing myself to travel gently into the future also keeps me from spending too much time in the past.

I have mostly moved on from agonizing about my many mistakes and humiliations. But a toxic cloud of self-judgment still gathers around me when I think about the faulty perceptions and beliefs that ruled my life for so long.

Why did I believe so fervently that alcohol was my friend? That having a social life was synonymous with drinking? That being unable to quit meant I was a loser who lacked strength, character, and willpower? How could what I thought was undisputed truth turn out to be so false?

Lately, though, I find I have banked enough self-compassion to explore these questions without beating up my past self quite so badly. I have found the emotional bandwidth to ask how I can support her from the present, where my feet are planted firmly on the ground—no longer pounding the endless treadmill.

And I have gained trust that some questions can't be answered intellectually. They arrive organically when my mind is quiet, and I can listen to the deepest parts of myself. We can't think our way out of everything. We must trust the compass of our intuition.

I want to share with you a final set of affirmations I wrote to help calibrate my inner compass, the one that keeps me oriented toward my intention. The better I am at recognizing the people and experiences that fill me up, the more easily I can find them. My expectations for how and when that happens is something I have learned to hold lightly.

> *I release all fear of missed opportunities.*
>
> *The more closely I listen to myself, the more clarity I receive.*
>
> *I am magnetic to people and experiences that fill me up.*
>
> *Every day, I make choices that lead me to the life I desire.*

As you calibrate your compass and embark on your new beginning, I want to tell you one last thing.

It is entirely possible for you to live a life that excites you and makes you thankful every day that you are fully present to experience it. Being present hurts a lot of the time, but the pain of living honestly and nakedly is beautiful in the possibilities it holds.

It teaches us that new growth almost always requires breaking open protective shells that once felt safe, sturdy, and comfortable.

It stretches the boundaries of our emotional universe, making room for new dimensions of joy and love.

It reveals to us our capacity to endure, thrive, and create.

It reminds us that we are alive.

ACKNOWLEDGMENTS

There are many people I want to thank for their contributions to this book and their support of me while I wrote it.

Laura Petersen, thank you for your guidance and accountability as I fought to complete this project. I honestly doubted at times if I could do it, but you never did, and for that I am so grateful.

To Keon Dillon, Leanne Naramore, Eliza Bean, and Amelia Jones, thank you for reading early versions of this work and lending me your expertise. I am honored to share the mycelium with you.

Kate Tomas, I hope you see your imprint on every page of this book. Your mentorship allowed me to trust my own mind in ways I never have before, and I can't thank or credit you enough for being my introduction to energy mastery.

Dina Kaplan and Marjorie Jean Kirkland, thank you for helping me develop the skills I needed to help other people incorporate yoga and meditation into their recoveries.

Erin Ranta, you taught me so much about the miracles and realities of recovery. I'm so proud to have had the opportunity to work with and learn from you.

To the amazing students of REVA, thank you for trusting me with your stories and your time. It is my honor to be a part of your journeys.

Chris Lanphear and Charles Kelly, thank you for giving me platform to explore my voice and for making the audiobook version of *Big Sober Energy* a reality.

I want to thank the many friends who stuck with me through the years, despite being somewhat hard to stick with at times. Big love to my crew from Grinnell College, the Eugene folks (especially the Emerald City Roller Girls and the Stitch-n-Bitchers), my SPLC family, the Wild Womyn of Alabama (and beyond), the Quaranteam of Jersey City, and JC West.

Lauryn Mascareñaz, Lindsay Bradley, Joanna Williams, and Monita Bell, thank you for believing in me as an author. Your faith means so much to me.

Thank you to my wonderful sisters, Anneke and Annalies, and their husbands, Ryan and Brendan, who have always been my cheerleaders.

To Mom and Dad, part of why I was able to make the difficult changes I needed to make and go on to write about them is the emotional safety and support you've always provided me. It is testimony to your parenting that you will be proud of me for writing a book, even though I'm sure the subject matter of this particular book may, at times, cause you to roll your eyes. ☺

Russell, it would have been impossible for me to accomplish this without your creativity, partnership, and unfailing love. Not only did you put up with me while I was still drinking, you've supported every direction I've expanded in my recovery—from starting podcasts to launching new businesses to writing books. It's not enough to say that, when it comes to men, you're "one of the good ones." You are a truly remarkable human, and I could not be more grateful for your patience, humor, love, and support.

APPENDICES

THREE THINKERS (OF MANY) WHO HAVE INFLUENCED ME

I have been wading in the waters of addiction literature for years now, and so many people have influenced my thinking on this topic. You'll find some of their work referenced in this book. But there are a few people whose names I want to share with you because their work has shaped my beliefs about the intersection of recovery and community and about what it means to be free in the Western World in the 21st century.

Explore them for yourself. Read them and support their work. It might contain the mind bombs you need to break down whatever walls exist between you, a community that needs your magic, and a future that feels like home.

Sonya Renee Taylor

Sonya Renee Taylor is a writer, spoken-word artist, activist, and public intellectual (among many other things) who wrote a life-changing book called *The Body Is Not an Apology: The Power of Radical Self-Love*. I say life-changing because I dare you to read it and not feel different afterward–about yourself, the people around you, and the systems we live within.

You've probably already come across the term *body terrorism* in Chapter 7. As far as I know, this term originated with Taylor, and she defines it as "the historical and contemporary violence associated with body hatred."[30]

Body terrorism occurs whenever a person's body is policed, jailed, abused, judged, or killed simply for existing. Slavery and lynching are body terrorism. Unfortunately, our society has historically tolerated these acts and continues to tolerate many forms of body terrorism today.

Consider these everyday acts of physical and psychological violence and control:

- Trying to "convert" gay youth by subjecting them to torment and humiliation.

- Posting nude photos of women online without their consent.

- Separating migrant children from their parents and putting them in cages.

- Jailing Black and Brown people for drug crimes while their white counterparts get probation and treatment.

- Denying life-saving social benefits to people with disabilities if they choose to get married.

- Forcing a 10-year-old to carry the baby of her rapist to full-term.

This concept resonated so strongly with me because one of the major blocks I had to overcome in sobriety was facing up to the war I had waged on my body while drinking and using. Except in my case, I viewed myself as the terrorist. The call was coming from inside the house.

But reading Taylor's book laid out in black and white the fact that self-inflicted harm is almost always a symptom of internalized hatred, and that hatred came from *outside* the house. She flipped the script on my culpability. She also flipped on a light, illuminating a dark room I thought I had been inhabiting alone. Looking around, I finally saw that my attacks on my body (plus the external attacks I'd become numb to over the years) connected me to every other person whose body is under attack, no matter where they live and breathe.

The conditions that compelled me to forego health and safety for the privilege of pouring booze into an unfillable void are the same conditions that cause humans to wreak havoc on one another's health and safety: judgment, bias, bigotry, consumerism, classism, nationalism, and every other manner of manufactured hierarchy, competition, and scarcity.

The isolation, the anxiety, and the fear caused by this artificial rendering of our humanity are the same. Some of us turn it on ourselves. Some of us turn it on others. Some of us do both. But all of us are diminished by it–even those we consider beneficiaries of the resulting systems of power.

My struggle is not the same struggle as a Black trans woman's, but as long as Black trans women are physically and psychologically unsafe, I am also unsafe, and so are you.

As long as bodies are policed and jailed and judged and valued unequally, we all–by definition–live in an unjust system. That's depressing, but you shouldn't let it defeat you, and Sonya Renee Taylor is here to tell you why: As long as you can carve out a zone of freedom within the roughly two cubic feet you occupy on this earth, you are doing something radical that fundamentally disrupts that system. The pathway to achieving the zone of freedom is radical self-love.

Self-love can be an activating concept for some people. Some days it might feel unachievable, especially if you belong to one or more marginalized groups. But like everything else in this book, it is something you can grow with intention and practice. The juice is so worth the squeeze. I require all my students to buy and read *The Body Is Not an Apology*, and I encourage you to buy and read it too. (Seriously, go do it!)

When you dare to love yourself abundantly in a society that wants you to stay quiet, obedient, and small, you accomplish two things.

One, you create freedom for yourself that no one can take away from you. When you own who you are, someone else's wish to diminish you no longer has the same impact. You may still experience body terrorism, but *you will no longer be an accomplice to the attacks!*

And two, you give other people permission to do the same. You become a force for unity and connection rather than a cog in the trauma machine that divides us.

Gabor Maté

Gabor Maté is a physician and writer whose work on addiction and trauma is helping to slowly chip away at narratives and beliefs that separate "addicts" from "normal" people. Instead, he asks us to look at addiction as a symptom of society.

I first became aware of Maté when my friend and business partner, Erin Ranta, recommended I read *In the Realm of Hungry Ghosts*. This book both complicates and simplifies addiction. I'd never heard anyone express in such depth and detail the idea that addiction is a continuum of experiences based on factors both cultural and neurological. By superimposing a strictly medical model on addiction treatment, says Maté, we distance ourselves from holistic solutions that could potentially heal us at the social level.

That part sounds complicated. But in our attempts to categorize and label each other, we've been collectively overlooking the simple part: Pathologizing people's experiences interferes with their self-understanding, and without self-understanding, recovery is almost impossible.

In other words, the way we talk about addiction is actually making it harder to recover. But if we can change our collective understanding, and study the nuances of how our physical and emotional predispositions interact with our social contexts, we can begin to reckon with the realities of how our society drives so many of us into the hell of addiction.

If *In the Realm of Hungry Ghosts* is one of the first mainstream books that opened the door to talking about how Western life creates the conditions for addiction, Maté's new book *The Myth of Normal* (co-written with his son Daniel) dives deep into how our increasingly isolated lives, combined with the pressures of capitalism, negatively affect almost every aspect of our health. In a recent interview on *Democracy Now!*, Maté shared the following thoughts (which were subsequently viewed 800,000 times on Instagram):

> *Most of us, because of the nature of the culture, the way we raise children, the way we have to relate to each other, the very values of a society are traumatizing for a lot of people. So, it's false to say that some people are normal and others are abnormal. In fact, we're all on a spectrum of woundedness, which has a great impact on how we relate to each other and our health....*
>
> *In a society that tells you that you're not enough, that you're not good enough, that you don't look good enough, that you don't have enough, that you don't own enough, that you haven't attained enough–creating a sense of emptiness is the fuel that runs the consumer society where never is there enough. You always have to have more and more....*
>
> *So basically, it's a highly addictive culture that feeds off people's addiction to drive its profits, and they do so quite deliberately. So this society runs on people's sense of deficient emptiness, where more and more is what they think is needed to fill that hole inside themselves.*[31]

The biggest thing I take away from Maté's work is that addiction is inevitable within a culture that values individuals over the collective, isolates families, and fetishizes wealth above all else. Capitalism teaches us to be addicted from birth. Without mitigating these pressures and changing our priorities, we are looking for solutions in the wrong places.

Again, this might seem depressing, but I find it hopeful. People in recovery are superheroes in my opinion. If we can take some of the self-understanding we've fought for and bring it out into the world, into our families, and into our communities, if we can start to intentionally subvert the narrative that *more* is always the answer, I believe we have the potential to spare others some of the pain we've experienced.

People with substance use disorders don't need to be curtained off and studied as a subset of afflicted individuals. We need to be listened to and seen and welcomed as members of every community. Our recoveries should be celebrated because, frankly, we are miracles. People around us need to know that. And those who are struggling need to know they are not alone.

Caroline Collado

The last person I want to mention is Caroline Collado, a writer, coach, speaker, and activist who identifies as an Afro-Taino, queer, non-binary, neurodivergent human in recovery from substance use issues. I first got to know Caroline's work via Instagram, where they post under the name of their platform, Recovery for the Revolution.

The first writing of Collado's I ever read was posted on January 12, 2021, under a graphic that read, "We can stay sober through the revolution." I won't quote the whole caption, but I still remember the pieces that stopped me in my tracks.

Recovery for the Revolution is just about this: How can we start and stay on our paths of recovery, whatever they may look like for us, while we go through major shifts and transitions socially, politically, environmentally, economically, and spiritually, and how can we bring about ways of being through our recovery that free us from the systems of oppression?...

> We need to be well. We must take care of ourselves. We must support each other through the shifts that are happening as we reckon with the unaddressed legacy of colonization, capitalism, white supremacy, patriarchy, and ableism that make people feel they cannot be in this planet and numb out/potentially risk death using substances and other coping mechanisms that are damaging to ourselves and others....[32]

After January 12, 2021, I became an avid reader of Collado's posts and blog. What hooked me and keeps me coming back is the clarity of their message, which I attempt to summarize here:

Our current systems are making us sick.

The people most exploited and harmed by our systems get the sickest.

Most of our recovery options are shaped by these same systems.

Thus, most recovery options fail the most vulnerable among us.

For this to change, the people pushed furthest to the margins by our current systems must be at the center of our new recovery paradigms!

Their primary call to action is to decolonize recovery spaces. If decolonization is a new term for you, this definition from the authors of the Racial Equity Tools website is helpful: "Shifting power towards political, economic, educational, cultural, psychic independence and power that originates from a colonized nation's own Indigenous culture."

Collado is issuing a wake-up call: Without doing the work of decolonizing recovery, we can't recover the many things that harm us about our culture, including the deep wounds that have been with us since our founding. Recovery for the revolution is not a metaphor. *We need to be well.*

At the time of publication, Collado is writing a book based on their work called *Answering the Call of the Ancestors.* I can't wait to read it, and I encourage you to as well. Theirs is a voice the world—not just the recovery world—needs to hear.

ADDITIONAL RESOURCES

RECOVERY RESOURCES

The resources I've listed here are a small selection taken from the growing number of options for people who either cannot or do not wish to participate in AA or pursue traditional treatment pathways. As I've said many times in this book, *I make no claim to know what is best for you or for anyone.* My goal is to shine a light on alternatives I wish I'd known about during the bleakest points in my struggle.

Big Sober Energy Community, Mentorship, and Courses

A small-group membership program and online courses based on the practices in this book, led by yours truly! *(bigsoberenergy.com)*

The Booze Breakup

A self-study and community program led by recovery coach Beth Bowen, who also hosts the *Sober Stories* podcast. *(bethbowen.co/booze-breakup-online-course)*

The Luckiest Club

An online membership community founded by Laura McKowen, author of *We Are the Luckiest*. *(theluckiestclub.com)*

Sober Mom Squad

Formed during the onset of the COVID-19 pandemic, SMS is an online membership and coaching community for mothers seeking support to stay sober through connection and mutual support. *(sobermomsquad.com)*

Sober Powered

A podcast with accompanying ebooks, online courses, and membership options, all created by sober scientist Gil Tietz. *(soberpowered.com)*

Recovery Dharma

A free alternative to AA that uses "Buddhist practices and principles to recover from addiction." *(recoverydharma.org)*

Tempest Sobriety School

A membership-based program and foundations course built using evidence-based treatment methods. *(jointempest.com)*

This Naked Mind

Based on author Annie Grace's widely-loved quit lit book of the same title, This Naked Mind offers both paid and no-cost options for learning her suggested "control alcohol" techniques. *(thisnakedmind.com)*

QUIT LIT AND OTHER RECOMMENDED RECOVERY BOOKS

There are so many amazing quit lit books out there, and more are being published all the time as the stigma around substance use disorders slowly shrinks. This is just a small sampling of titles that inspired me and switched on lightbulbs of empowerment and self-recognition in early sobriety.

Whenever possible, please buy through independent or Black-owned booksellers. If you shop online, consider using bookshop.org over Amazon.

Alcohol Lied to Me: How to Stop Drinking and Get the Real You Back by Craig Beck

A self-development book based on the experiences of a stereotypically successful man who denied his problem drinking for over two decades. This is one of the first recovery books I ever read, and it helped me recognize that alcohol wasn't the best friend I thought it was.

Blackout: Remembering the Things I Drank to Forget by Sarah Hepola

I have read this book at least three times, and I never re-read books. It is my favorite quit lit read. Sarah's drinking experiences and mine don't align completely, but the inner struggle she experienced after having blackouts and finally accepting the need to get sober resonated with me as clearly as a bell.

The Craving Mind: From Cigarettes to Smartphones to Love— Why We Get Hooked and How We Can Break Bad Habits by Dr. Jud Brewer

An evidence-based look at the mechanism of craving and how mindfulness can help, engagingly told by an academic with personal experience as both clinician and patient. I reference this book almost daily in my own life and recommend it to all my students.

First in the Family by Jessica Hoppe

To quote *Publisher's Marketplace Deal Report*, *First in the Family* is "a memoir chronicling the author's recovery, deconstructing American exceptionalism and whiteness within powerful institutions such as AA, and reconciling the personal, familial, historical, and political to interrupt cycles of harm."

In the Realm of Hungry Ghosts: Close Encounters With Addiction by Gabor Maté

A breakthrough title in the recovery genre about the roots of addiction and how our social, political, and medical institutions consistently fail people with substance use disorders. Required reading for anyone who has ever felt like we are all collectively missing something. Spoiler alert: WE ARE.

Quit Like a Woman: The Radical Choice to Not Drink in a Culture Obsessed with Alcohol by Holly Whitaker

Part memoir, part nonfiction reporting, this book offers a deep dive into the history of Big Alcohol, the problematic origins of AA, and connections between substance use disorders and social justice. Holly also writes a valuable Substack blog called Recovering and co-hosts a podcast with Emily McDowell called *Quitted*.

Recovering the Home by Jocellyn Snyder (neé Harvey)

This book is no longer widely available, which is why I am so thrilled that Jocellyn has generously given *Big Sober Energy* readers access to it. As outlined in Chapter 12, *Recovering the Home* is a practical guide to remaking your living space to align with your post-alcohol life. You can download this book for free at **bigsoberenergy.com/reader-bonuses.**

The Red Road to Wellbriety: In the Native American Way by White Bison

A recovery book by and for Native American people who wish to access and integrate Indigenous wisdom in their recovery journeys. The book references the 12 steps of AA but offers them in a holistic, nature-based context.

The Sober Lush: A Hedonist's Guide to Living a Decadent, Adventurous, Soulful Life—Alcohol Free by Amanda Eyre Ward and Jardine Libaire

A self-development book encouraging readers to view sober life as a gift, an adventure, and even an opportunity to explore hedonism.

Sunshine Warm Sober: The Unexpected Joy of Being Sober— Forever by Catherine Gray

A memoir sprinkled with interviews about a single woman's experience of "what comes next?" after she makes it through early sobriety. I also recommend Catherine's first book, *The Unexpected Joy of Being Sober*, about her early sobriety.

We Are the Luckiest: The Surprising Magic of a Sober Life by Laura McKowen

Essays about a single mother's sobriety journey, including lessons and suggestions about recovering one's identity and self-worth.

SPIRITUALITY AND YOGA RESOURCES

I hesitated to include this list because everyone's journey is so personal, and the universe of such books, podcasts, and teachers is seemingly endless. However, these are a handful of resources I either lean on heavily myself or find myself recommending over and over, so here they are.

Love and Rage: The Path of Liberation Through Anger by Lama Rod Owens

This book isn't explicitly about substance use disorder, but the subject of how to live with and make use of anger while still pursuing a free life holds incredible value for people on a recovery journey. Rod Owens is also one of my favorite teachers to watch on YouTube.

Mindfulness in Plain English by Henepola Gunaratana

I reference this book constantly. Not only is it an accessible introduction to vipassana meditation and Buddhist wisdom, but the writing is a joy, and I learn something new every time I flip through its pages.

Recovery Dharma: How to Use Buddhist Practices and Principles to Heal the Suffering of Addiction

This is the primary text of the Recovery Dharma program, and the title pretty much says it all. The book is available for free online at recoverydharmanyc.org under the resources tab.

Rev. angel Kyodo williams

Rev. williams is an African-American Zen Buddhist priest, spiritual teacher, visionary leader, and author of the books *Radical Dharma: Talking Race, Love, and Liberation* and *Being Black: Zen and the Art of Living With Fearlessness and Grace.* Among many other accomplishments, she regularly gathers a rich online community of justice-oriented practitioners who meditate together regularly. (angelkyodowilliams.com)

Taylor Hunt

Taylor is an Ashtanga yoga teacher in long-term recovery from heroin addiction. He has committed his life and career to helping others deepen their healing through an intentional and traditional yoga practice. You can find his instructional videos for free on Vimeo. (taylorhuntyoga.com)

Yoga Is Dead podcast by Tejal Patel and Jesal Parikh

A fascinating six-episode podcast exploring the many ways modern yoga studios and teachers undermine the original spiritual teachings that brought yoga into being. Each episode includes a detailed resource list for further exploration. (yogaisdeadpodcast.com)

SELECTED SPIRITUAL TEXTS

Translations of key, original, primary-source Buddhist and Hindu texts available for free online at the time of publication. Many of the concepts related to universal divine energy and collective consciousness outlined in this book originated in these texts.

The Vedas

This is an open-source translation of four texts widely believed to be the original scriptures of Hinduism. *(bit.ly/four-vedas)*

- *The Rigveda*
- *The Yajurveda*
- *The Samaveda*
- *The Atharvaveda*

Other Early Hindu Texts

Open source translations of two additional early Hindu texts frequently referenced and cited in spiritual teaching and literature.

- **The Early Upanisads (bit.ly/early-upanisads)**
- **The Bhagavad Gita (bit.ly/free-bhagavad-gita)**

All About Hinduism

An introduction to Hinduism, including various aspects of Hindu philosophy, theology, symbols, rituals, and scriptures, among other illuminating details. *(bit.ly/all-about-hinduism)*

Sutra Central

A website bringing together translations of the Tipiṭaka or "Three Baskets" of Buddhist wisdom. These texts are believed to be the direct teachings of the Buddha himself or of his disciples. *(suttacentral.net)*

MORE RECOMMENDED READING

A selection of titles I recommend to my students and anyone else who will listen.

Whenever possible, please buy through independent or Black-owned booksellers. If you wish to buy online, consider using bookshop.org over Amazon.

The Body Is Not an Apology and *Your Body is Not an Apology* by Sonya Renee Taylor

The Body Keeps the Score: Brain, Mind, and Body in the Healing of Trauma by Bessel van der Kolk

Disability Visibility: First-Person Stories from the Twenty-First Century by Alice Wong

The Feel Good Effect: Reclaim Your Wellness by Finding Small Shifts that Create Big Change by Robyn Conley Downs

The Myth of Normal: Trauma, Illness, and Healing in a Toxic Culture by Gabor Maté

Self-Compassion: The Proven Power of Being Kind to Yourself by Kristin Neff

BIG SOBER ENERGY READER BONUSES

This book is for you, and my most sincere wish is that you feel empowered to use it. To make it as simple as possible for you to integrate these energy practices into your life, I've linked helpful resources throughout the book that add scaffolding or offer you the opportunity to deepen your learning.

All the resources linked throughout the book are listed here by chapter. I've also gathered them in one place at **bigsoberenergy.com/ reader-bonuses.** Simply enter your email to access the resource landing page. You can bookmark that page and come back to it whenever you need it. (I'll send you the link via email as well.)

This list is a work in progress; I'll keep you updated whenever I improve an existing resource or add something new!

Chapter 1
Recovery blog post: "Hi. I'm Adrienne, and I'm Sober."

Chapter 5
Article for *Spirituality & Health*: "Mindfulness Over Merlot"

Chapter 6
Recovery blog post: "Hi. I'm Adrienne, and I'm Sober."

EFT audio recording: Affirmations for Self-Trust and Forgiveness

Chapter 10
Guided visualization audio recording: Energy Center Visualization

Chapter 12
Feminist Hotdog podcast interview with Jocellyn Harvey: "Feminism and Sobriety, Part III"

Recovering the Home by Jocellyn Snyder (neé Harvey)

Chapter 13
Feminist Hotdog podcast interview with Holly Whitaker: "Feminism and Sobriety, Part I"

Feminist Hotdog podcast interview with Cynthia Wright: "Getting Your Sh*t Together with Cynthia Wright"

Chapter 14
Feminist Hotdog podcast interview with Dr. Kate Tomas: "Radical Magick"

Chapter 15
Guided meditation audio recording: Metta Meditation for People in Recovery

Feminist Hotdog podcast interview with Jessica Hoppe: "Racism and Recovery"

Chapter 16
Getting Started: Creating Your Plan worksheet

CHAPTERS AT A GLANCE

CHAPTER	BENEFITS	ELEMENT
MINDFUL ENERGY: NAVIGATING YOURSELF		
Chapter 5: How Do I Feel?	Self-Awareness, Emotional Regulation	**INTENTION:** Notice your feelings. **MEDITATION:** Commit to a daily practice. **ALIGNED ACTION:** RAIN **INTEGRATION:** Activate your parasympathetic nervous system. Learn about the brain science of cravings.
Chapter 6: Self-Compassion v. Shame	Confidence, Self-Trust, Self-Compassion	**INTENTION:** Prioritize your relationship with yourself. **MEDITATION:** Opening to Self meditation **ALIGNED ACTION:** EFT with affirmations for self-trust and forgiveness **INTEGRATION:** Craft an energetically aligned apology.
Chapter 7: Body and Soul	Stress Reduction, Confidence, Emotional Regulation	**INTENTION:** Embrace the deliberate nature of healing. **MEDITATION:** Walking meditation **ALIGNED ACTION:** Self massage, goddess pose, legs up the wall **INTEGRATION:** EFT with affirmations for anxiety, singing and laughing, dancing

CHAPTER	BENEFITS	ELEMENT
Chapter 8: Truth Be Told	Integrity, Stress Relief, Positive Connection	**INTENTION:** Commit to telling the truth all the time. **MEDITATION:** Say affirmations for truth-telling. Visualize lies leaving your life. **ALIGNED ACTION:** Pick your parameters. Notice your patterns. Turn the honesty inward. **INTEGRATION:** Honesty is its own form of integration; if you find a difficult truth coming up, consider working through it with a therapist.
ENERGY BOUNDARIES: NAVIGATING OTHER PEOPLE		
Chapter 9: What Makes Me Happy?	Emotional Regulation, Self-Advocacy	**INTENTION:** Notice what makes you happy. **MEDITATION:** Commit to a daily practice. Visualize a desirable outcome. **ALIGNED ACTION:** Life Edit (Obligation Inventory) **INTEGRATION:** Make "no" your default answer. Never agree to anything in the moment.
Chapter 10: How to Plug an Energy Leak	Positive Connection, Self-Advocacy, Time Management, Stress Reduction	**INTENTION:** Grow your power. Identify energy vampires. Differentiate your energy from others'. **MEDITATION:** Energy center visualization **ALIGNED ACTION:** Rolling up the window, body scan and cord cutting, mirror suit **INTEGRATION:** Make meaning, then let it go.

CHAPTER	BENEFITS	ELEMENT
Chapter 11: Happy Place or Hellscape?	Time Management, Stress Reduction, Emotional Regulation	**INTENTION:** Ask yourself, "Why am I on social media?" **MEDITATION:** Micro-meditation, RAIN, belly breathing **ALIGNED ACTION:** Use a time-limiting app. Get your phone out of your bedroom. Set a scrolling date. Employ "latergram." Don't read the comments. **INTEGRATION:** Revisit your "why" and your relationship with social media regularly. Assess its value on an ongoing basis.
PRACTICAL ENERGY: NAVIGATING THE WORLD		
Chapter 12: Recovering Your Home	Organization, Emotional Regulation, Stress Reduction	**INTENTION:** Assess how you feel and how you want to feel about your space. **MEDITATION:** Mindfully observe your emotions as you look at your things. **ALIGNED ACTION:** Sort your belongings as either "keep," "give," or discard." Personalize your sober space. **INTEGRATION:** Reflect on the sorting process. Shop mindfully going forward.
Chapter 13: What's in the Box?	Organization, Time Management, Stability, Stress Reduction, Confidence	**INTENTION:** Focus on gradual, incremental progress. Take getting your shit together seriously. **MEDITATION:** Visualize your life without disorder and chaos. **ALIGNED ACTION:** Schedule, automate, outsource, and rely on robots. **INTEGRATION:** Reward yourself. Get organized with friends.

CHAPTER	BENEFITS	ELEMENT
Chapter 14: Banish the Money Monster	Financial Stability, Confidence, Stress Reduction, Self-Compassion	**INTENTION:** Establish a new energetic relationship with money. **MEDITATION:** Identify your money stories. **ALIGNED ACTION:** Face the money monster. Reimagine the nature of money. **INTEGRATION:** Be deliberate if you have a money meltdown.
Chapter 15: Chasing the Gleam	Positive Connection, Purpose, Fulfillment	**INTENTION:** Show up as who you are. Accept others for who they are. **MEDITATION:** Metta or Loving Kindness **ALIGNED ACTION:** Find your sober community. **INTEGRATION:** Collapse the hierarchy in your head. Expand your definition of community to everyone experiencing substance use disorder.

WORKS CITED OR CONSULTED

1   "Does AA Really Work?" *Into Action Recovery Centers.* Accessed 23 December 2022.

2   "What Is Sankalpa?" *Eshwar Bhakti.* Accessed 21 November 2022.

3   Gleeson, Jessamy. "Explainer: What Does Gaslight Mean?" *The Conversation,* 5 December, 2018.

4   Francis, Matthew. "Eight Things You Might Not Know About Light." *Symmetry Magazine,* 19 April 2016.

5   Gunaratana, Henepola. *Mindfulness in Plain English.* Wisdom Publications, 2002, pp. 3-4.

6   Ibid, p. 4.

7   Gray, Catherine. *Sunshine Warm Sober.* Octopus Books, 2021, pp. 245-246.

8   Frawley, David. "Understanding Prana." *Yoga International.* Accessed 21 December 2022.

9   Vallance, J.T. "Pneuma." *Oxford Classical Dictionary,* 7 March 2016.

10 Frantzis, Bruce. "What Is Chi?" *Energy Arts,* 15 April 2011.

11 "What Does Ki Mean, and How It Is Used in Japanese." *Japanese Universe,* 4 March 2022.

12 Frager, Robert. "Your Seven Souls: A Sufi View." *The Theosophical Society in America.* Accessed 21 December 2022.

13 "The Theory of Tibetan Medicine." *Aurora Tibetan Medicine.* Accessed 14 December 2022.

14 "What Is Mana?" *Mānoa Heritage Center.* Accessed 14 December 2022.

15 "Nwyfre." Emrys y Dewin, 20 March 2019.

16 Cascio, Christopher N., et al. "Self-Affirmation Activates Brain Systems Associated with Self-Related Processing and Reward and Is Reinforced by Future Orientation." *Social Cognitive and Affective Neuroscience,* vol. 11, no. 4, 2016, pp. 621-9.

17 Jam, Rain. "The Ultimate Guide to Yin Yoga: Principles, Benefits & Misconceptions." *Arhanta Yoga Ashrams,* 15 September 2016.

18 "Original Yin." *Yin Yoga.* Accessed 21 November 2022.

19 Taylor, Sonya Renee. "What is Body Terrorism?" *The Body Is Not an Apology.* Accessed 18 December 2022.

20 "The Growing Popularity of Somatic Practices." *Omega.* Accessed 21 November 2022.

21 Kaplan, Dina. "Two Years to No Lies." *Medium.* Accessed 21 November 2022.

22   Wallace, Christopher. "The Real Story on the Chakras." *Hareesh Blog*, 5 February 2016.

23   Dean, Brian. "Instagram Demographic Statistics." *Backlinko*, 5 January 2022.

24   powell, john a. "Bridging and Breaking." *Othering & Belonging Institute at UC Berkeley*. Accessed 14 December 2022.

25   Hatchard, G D, et al. "Maharishi Effect: A Model for Social Improvement. Time Series Analysis of a Phase Transition to Reduced Crime in Merseyside Metropolitan Area." *Psychology, Crime & Law*, vol. 2, no. 3, 1996, pp. 165-174.

26   Barnhofer, Thorsten, et al. "State Effects of Two Forms of Meditation on Prefrontal EEG Asymmetry in Previously Depressed Individuals." *Mindfulness*, vol. 1, no. 1, 2010, pp. 21-27.

27   Hoppe, Jessica. "The First Step to Recovery Is admitting You Are Not Powerless Over Your Privilege." *GEN (Medium)*, 6 July 2020.

28   hill, myisha t. *Heal Your Way Forward: The Co-Conspirator's Guide to an Anti-racist Future.* Row House Publishing, 2022.

29   Rizvi, Saqib. "Manifestation Without Attachment." *Insight Timer*, August 2020.

30   Taylor, Sonya Renee. "What is Body Terrorism?" *The Body Is Not an Apology*. Accessed 18 December 2022.

31   "Dr. Gabor Maté on 'The Myth of Normal,' Healing in a Toxic Culture & How Capitalism Fuels Addiction." *Democracy Now*, 24 November 2022.

32   Collado, Carolyn. "We Can Stay in Recovery Through the Revolution." *Recovery for the Revolution*. Accessed 21 December 2022.

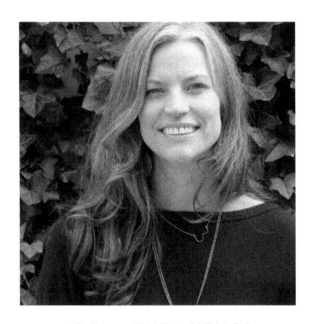

ABOUT THE AUTHOR

Adrienne van der Valk is an author, speaker, certified meditation and yoga teacher, co-host of *The Hangover Liberation Society* podcast, and founder of the Big Sober Energy community.

As a trauma-informed recovery mentor, Adrienne focuses on using meditation, movement, and energy mastery practices to help students align their minds and bodies with the sober lives they want. In addition to her formal training, Adrienne's mentorship framework draws on two decades of experience in social work and education, years of research on the neuroscience of addiction, her personal journey with alcohol use disorder, and the inspiring successes of her students.

Adrienne is also an activist who teaches, writes, and speaks about the connections between addiction and social justice. She holds a BA in sociology from Grinnell College and MS degrees in journalism and political science from the University of Oregon. She lives in Palm Springs, California, with her husband and a pit bull named Zola.

Printed in the USA
CPSIA information can be obtained
at www.ICGtesting.com
LVHW020245250924
791984LV00014B/333